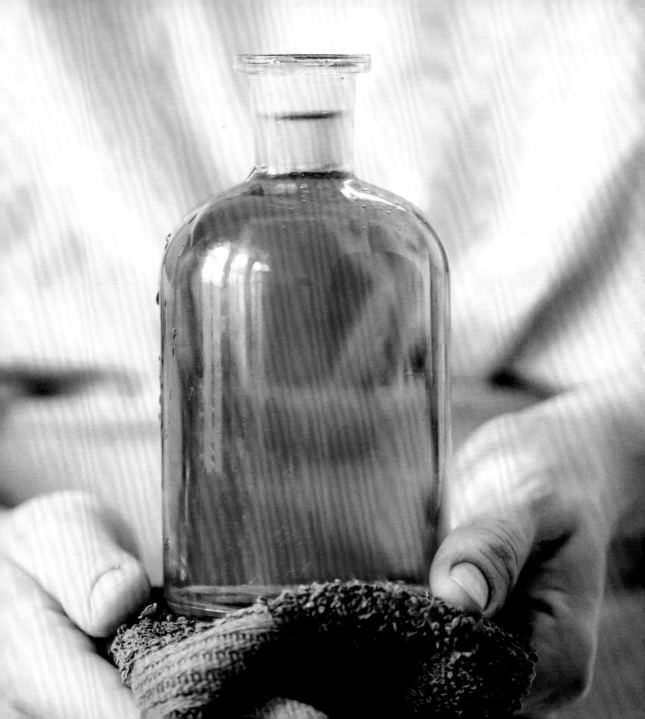

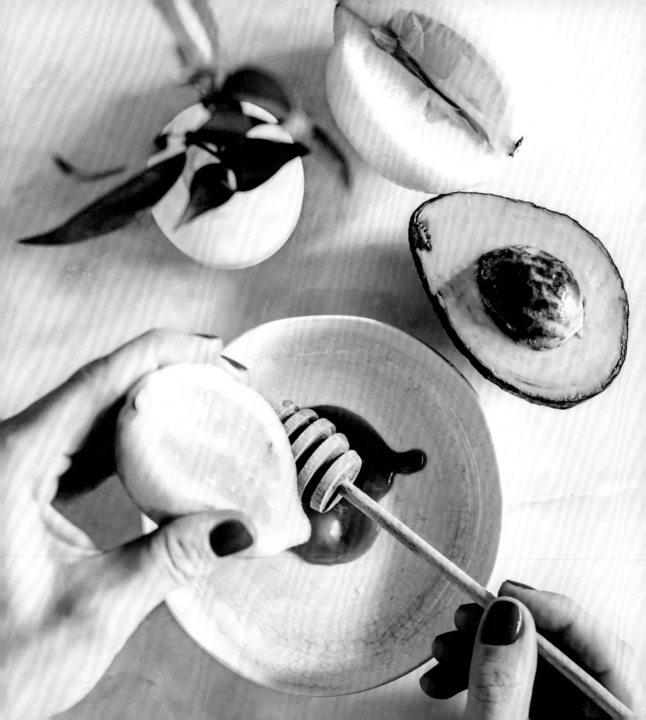

hello *gorgeous*

100 FABULOUS **DIY FACIALS**
YOU CAN DO AT HOME

STEPHANIE GERBER

weldon**owen**

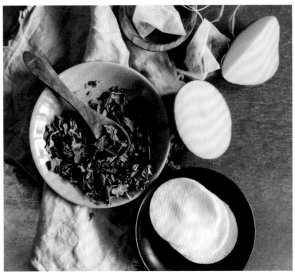
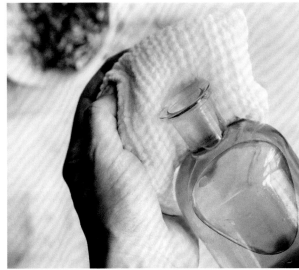

CONTENTS

PART ONE
EVERYDAY SKINCARE

CLEANSE

EXFOLIATE

TONERS & MISTS

EYE MASKS

LIP MASKS

SERUMS

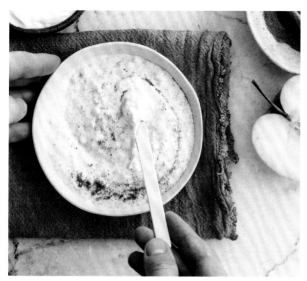
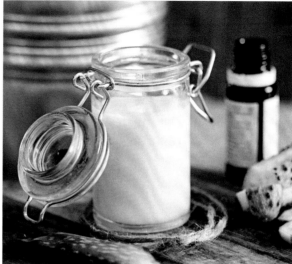

PART TWO

PERSONALIZE YOUR SKINCARE ROUTINE

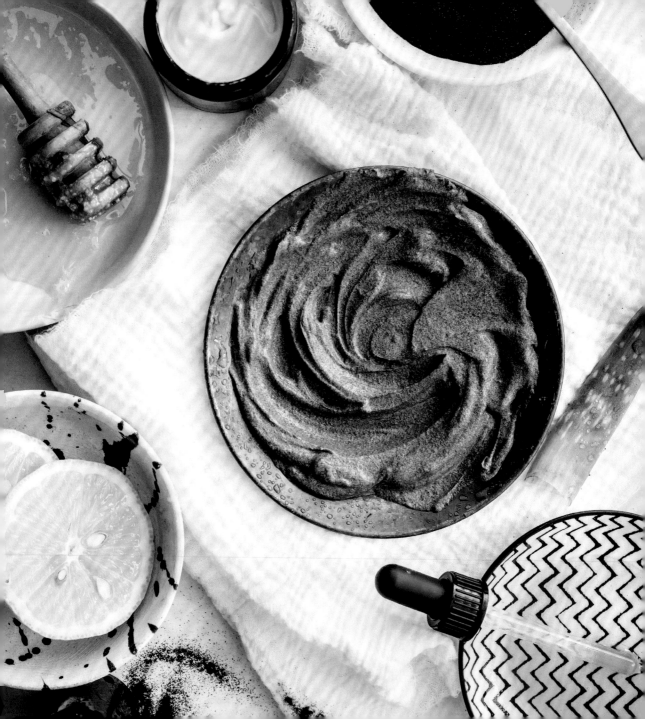

INTRODUCTION

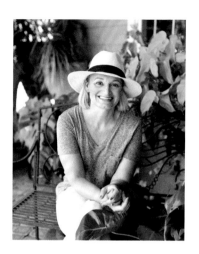

IF I HAD TO CHOOSE a favorite skincare product, it would definitely be face masks. Clay masks, honey masks, sheet masks, I love them all. They're the best way to get that fresh-from-the-spa glow at home—plus, when you've got a mask on your face, it gives you an excuse to spend 15 minutes with a good book (or a trashy reality show) and relax a little bit.

And when those 15 minutes are up? Your skin feels softer, your pores are tighter, and you feel fantastic, because the best thing about face masks is the quick, noticeable results you get from them.

It's safe to say this book has a face mask for everything: acne, uneven skin tone, aging skin, you name it! No matter your skin type, be it oily, dry, or somewhere in between, you can benefit from adding face masks to your skincare regimen. Because whatever the problem, it can probably be remedied the natural way: with nourishing food on your face. If it's good enough to eat, it's good enough to put on your face, right?

If you're looking to amp up your skincare self-care, doing so at home is not only convenient, but it also gives you the empowerment of knowing what you're putting on your face. So go ahead, we're giving you permission to raid the pantry. Yes, things can get messy, but your glowing skin will thank you!

Stephanie Gruber

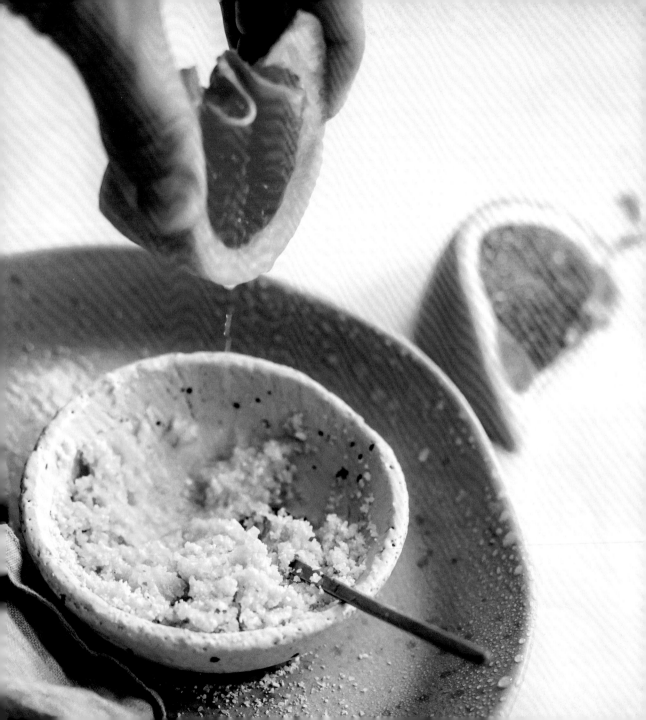

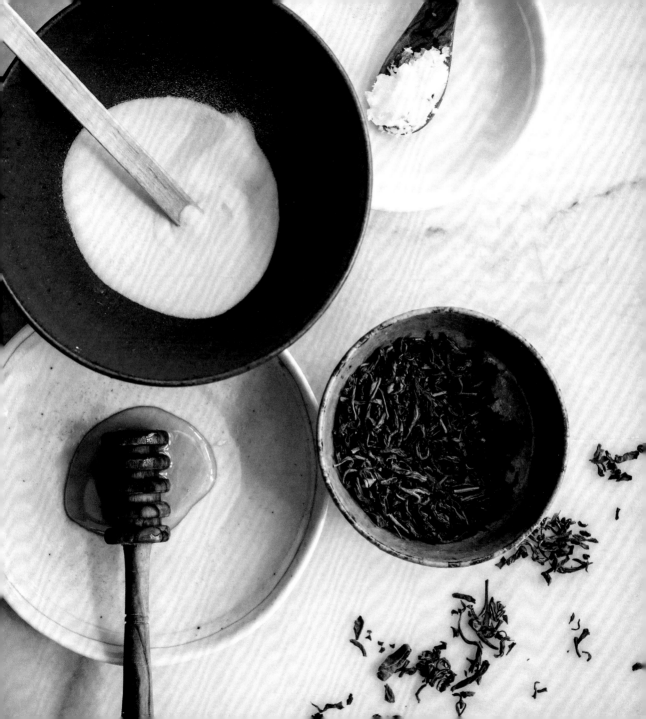

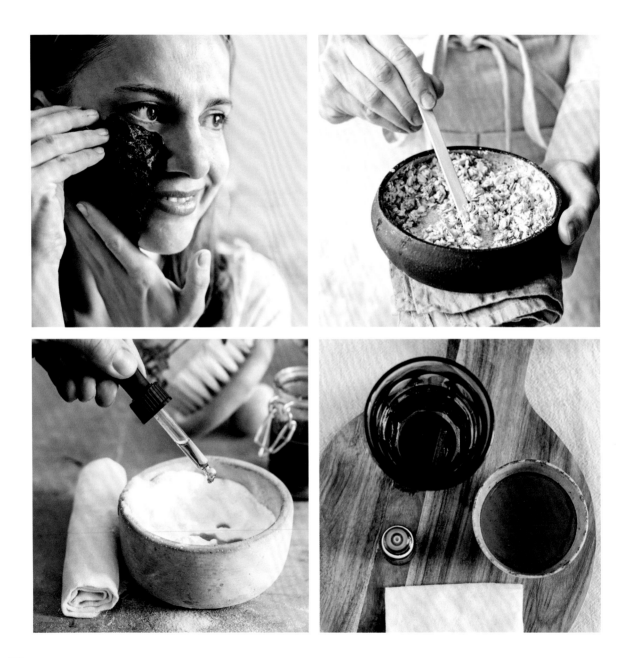

NATURAL BEAUTY BASICS

Face masks are not only good for your skin, they feel wonderful too—the best way to get that spa experience at home. So pamper yourself and your skin with the masks in this book, whatever your skin might need. Between the wonderful natural ingredients and the simple, effective results, you'll be left feeling gorgeous inside and out.

1

Picking the Mask
Face masks are wonderful in part because of how well they target specific issues, so keep that in mind when you pick your mask—whether it's exfoliating, hydrating, anti-aging, oil balancing, complexion brightening, or almost anything else.

2

Applying the Mask
Masks should always be applied to freshly cleansed skin, and can pretty much always be applied with either your fingertips or a facial brush. Usually, you'll want to keep a mask on for 10 to 20 minutes, but always check the directions to make sure you're getting the most out of the mask.

But don't use the same mask too often. Doing so too much can cause irritation and even sensitivities to certain ingredients. Definitely something to avoid. Go for 1 to 3 times a week instead, and save the other days for different masks.

3

After the Mask
Removing the mask with a warm washcloth helps not only thoroughly remove the mask off, but allows a little extra exfoliation. Always follow with a serum or moisturizer.

And then relax! Enjoy the feeling of having pampered yourself, and of the wonderful effects to come.

ASSEMBLING A TOOLKIT

Nothing makes me crazier than mixing a mask or toner, only to realize I forgot a basic tool. It took me an embarrassing amount of time to realize my life would be *much* easier if I just bought a set of dedicated DIY tools—which is surprisingly simple and inexpensive.

And worth it. Because there are only so many jam jars a family can go through, and trying to cook dinner with the same tools you just used for clay? Is not recommended.

Measuring cups
Pretty self-explanatory!

Measuring spoons
Avoid metal because you shouldn't use it with clay.

Mixing bowls
A set with lids is ideal for mixing face mask ingredients together and storing leftovers in the fridge. Again, go with glass—it just makes life easier.

Small blender
A small handheld or immersion blender quickly mixes and purees ingredients. Much easier than digging out the food processor!

Coffee grinder
It's unexpected, but invaluable. Mine gets used on the regular to grind almonds, rice, oatmeal, and dried herbs.

Funnel
There's nothing worse than trying to pour a concoction into a storage bottle and spilling half of it on the counter.

Small spray bottles
You have to have something to spritz those mists and toners onto your face.

Facial brush
Yes, you can definitely use your fingers. But trust me, this little tool makes applying masks much less messy.

Soft washcloth
Perfect for a quick steam before your mask to open up the pores. Also helpful for gently removing the mask without damaging skin.

Headband
Besides keeping your hair back, it'll make it easy to apply your mask up to your hairline, an often-neglected area.

STOCKING THE PANTRY

Homemade beauty products can be super simple—especially since so many remedies and recipes contain the same soothing ingredients. Load up on a few essential items, and you'll be prepared to whip up virtually any mask you desire.

Aloe vera
Aloe vera gel contains a plethora of amino acids, minerals, and vitamins that benefit your skin and hair. It's a tried-and-true remedy for sunburns and inflammation that moisturizes and soothes any skin type.

Clay
Natural clay has long been known for its ability to draw out oil and impurities, as well as tighten and tone your skin.

Honey
Honey is a panacea for any skin type, locking in moisture and regulating hydration without clogging pores. It's naturally antibacterial and antifungal, too. Look for raw, organic honey.

Oats
Oats can help regulate your skin's pH levels, relieve redness and itchiness, and help treat skin conditions. They also gently exfoliate, making them perfect for face masks.

Tea
White, green, and black teas contain powerful antioxidants that help combat sun damage by absorbing UV rays and free radicals, while also soothing skin.

Apple cider vinegar
Trusty ACV is full of natural hydroxy acids that gently exfoliate your skin. Applying organic ACV also delivers beneficial enzymes, proteins, and good bacteria for healthy rejuvenation.

Activated charcoal
Charcoal has an amazing ability to bind with impurities, so bacteria, dead cells, oil and toxins are swept away as soon as it enters the game.

Yogurt
Yogurt contains lactic acid that gently dissolves dead skin cells, unclogs pores, kills bacteria, and evens skin tone. Choose the plain kind without added fruit or sugar.

Witch hazel
This gentle miracle ingredient fights inflammation and regulates oil production, so it's perfect for anyone with oily or sensitive skin. Look for pure witch hazel that isn't diluted with skin-drying alcohol.

THE SIMPLEST RECIPES

One of the best parts of DIY beauty is how incredibly *simple* it can be, especially once you understand the breakdown of a basic recipe. While the rest of this book offers specific recipes—some simple, some less so—that have specific benefits, this chart shows you how to build and customize simple face masks, so you can make your own, perfectly tailored to you, whenever you like.

1 SKIN TYPE
Start by measuring out ¼ cup of one of the base ingredients, determined by your skin type.

OILY
BENTONITE CLAY

Clay is great at absorbing excess oil and impurities.

2 YOUR GOAL
So, why are you making this mask today? Figure out your goals , and stir in 1 tablespoon of the add-in that will help you get there.

REDUCE WRINKLES
JOJOBA OIL

Helps smooth fine lines and reverse the signs of aging.

3 ESSENTIAL OILS
Mood enhancement starts here! If you'd like, add 3 drops of an essential oil associated with how you'd like to feel when you apply this mask—and all day long!

HAPPY
FRANKINCENSE OIL

For feelings of joy and peace.

4 BONUS ACTION
Multitask that mask! If you'd like an additional booster, mix in 1 tablespoon of the following actives.

MINIMIZE SCARRING
PUREED PUMPKIN

A natural source of alpha hydroxy acids to dissolve dead skin cells.

SENSITIVE

ALOE VERA GEL

Aloe is a natural anti-infammatory acting to soothe irritated skin.

INFLAMMATION

HONEY

With its soothing properties, honey can calm skin and even relieve rashes.

SLEEPY

LAVENDER OIL

Perfect for an overnight or evening mask, lavender encourages restful sleep.

SHRINK PORES

APPLE CIDER VINEGAR

One of the first astringents used for beauty, and still one of the best.

DRY

COOKED OATMEAL

The Beta-glucans in this breakfast fave help seal in moisture.

TIGHTEN SKIN

EGG WHITES

The protein in egg whites tighten the skin making you feel firmer.

CALM

SANDALWOOD OIL

Has been shown to reduce blood pressure and increase relaxation.

BREAKOUTS

CINNAMON

An antibacterial, it fights the bacteria that cause acne.

COMBINATION

PLAIN YOGURT

Don't go non-fat here! The fats help moisture, while the lactic acid controls oil production.

PIGMENTATION

CHOPPED PARSLEY

Of course, there are stronger anti-dark spot acids out there, but parsley is gently on your skin.

ENERGIZED

SWEET ORANGE OIL

Gets your blood pumping and helps to clear toxins and your mind.

BRIGHTEN SKIN

MASHED STRAWBERRIES

Vitamin C is an antioxidant and natural exfoliant, and strawberries are rich in it.

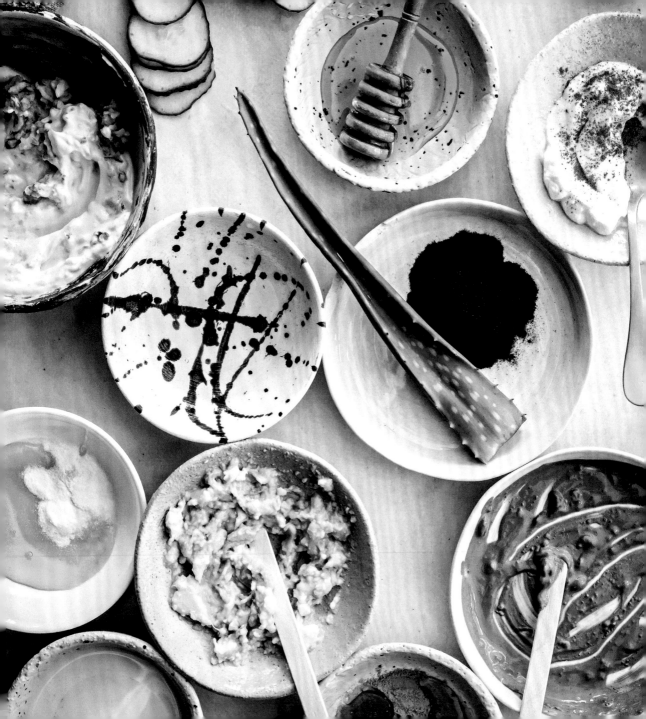

— Part 1 —

Everyday Skincare

Cleanse

Our skin accumulates makeup, dirt, and oil every day. It's one of the hazards of living in the world! Whether it's sweat, pollutants in the air, or oils coming from the fact that it's impossible to stop touching your face, stuff just gets on your face—and that's if you don't have kids with homemade craft projects. All that is why we cleanse our skin every night (right?!), but cleansers don't have to be soap based. You can lift away grime and clear out your pores without the harsh ingredients.

And that's where these masks step in. From toxin-absorbing charcoal to antibacterial honey to antioxidant-rich cinnamon, the ingredients in these masks will leave your skin supple and sparkling. Whichever mask you choose, you're in for a treat.

Activated Charcoal Cleanser

Charcoal is known for absorbing toxins internally—but it can also do so on the face, helping with fine particles and mild materials, this cleanser is a completely gentle mini-facial.

MATERIALS

2 tablespoons liquid Castile soap (preferably unscented, lavender, or another mild scent)

1 tablespoon almond oil (can also use jojoba, apricot kernel, or vitamin E oil)

2 tablespoons brown or white rice flour, finely ground

1 tablespoon baking soda

2 teaspoons activated charcoal

2 to 3 drops lavender essential oil (optional)

TOOLS

Coffee grinder

1 / In a small bowl, stir together the Castile soap and oil.

2 / Add the rice flour, baking soda, and activated charcoal. The mixture may bubble up a bit.

3 / Keep stirring until smooth and creamy. At this point, add the lavender essential oil, if using.

4 / Transfer the mixture to an airtight container and store it in a cool, dry place. If the scrub becomes dry, add a little water or almond oil and stir again until creamy.

5 / To use, splash face with a little water to make damp. Take 1 to 2 teaspoons of the cleanser and gently apply to the face with fingertips, using small, circular motions and being careful to avoid the area around the eyes.

6 / If desired, let the scrub sit on the face for a few minutes for extra oil-absorbing benefits.

7 / Rinse with lukewarm water and pat face dry. Follow with your favorite serum or moisturizer. For best results, use 2 to 3 times a week.

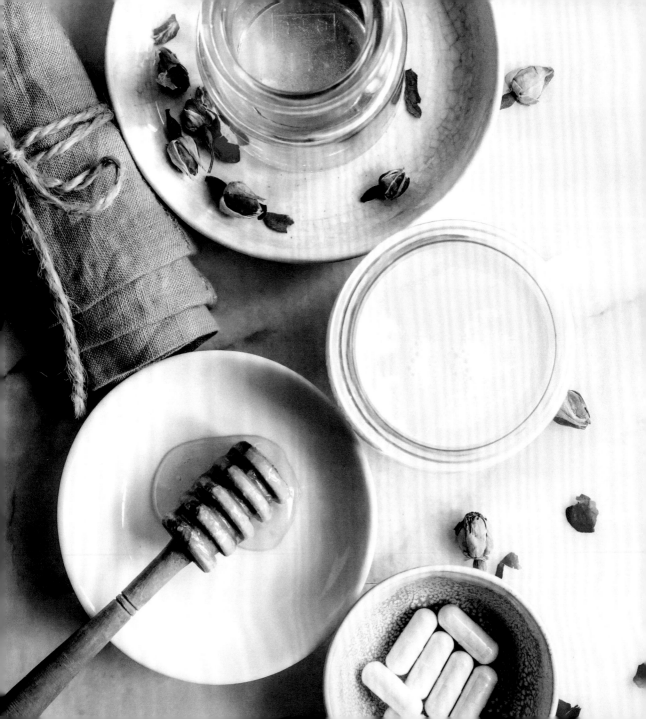

Probiotic Rose Milk Cleanser

You probably know the benefits of good bacteria for the gut—but they can help your skin too, by fighting harmful free radicals and reducing inflammation. Just use the same probiotics you would normally ingest! This recipe is perfect for skin that's prone to breakouts, but it's soothing and gentle enough for sensitive skin as well.

MATERIALS

1 teaspoon rosewater

1 tablespoon organic coconut milk from can

2 capsules live probiotics

1 tablespoon raw honey

TIP
If you want, you can substitute in coconut oil for coconut milk.

1 / Make your own rosewater using the recipe on page 53. For the coconut milk, be sure to scoop out the cream of the coconut milk, and not the watery liquid.

2 / Pour the coconut milk into a glass jar and add the rosewater.

3 / Add in the live probiotics and raw honey—itself loaded with probiotics! Stir thoroughly.

4 / Apply 1 to 2 teaspoons to your face and neck, massaging it in with slow, gentle circles for at least a minute before rinsing with warm water.

5 / Cover and store in the refrigerator to keep the bacteria active. To soften, warm the jar in the palms of your hands before use. For best results, use 2 to 3 times a week.

Apple + Cinnamon Cleansing Mask

This is a great mask for those with oily or acne-prone skin. The natural alpha hydroxy acid in the apples and the lactic acid in yogurt exfoliate the skin, while the oatmeal soothes inflammation. And cinnamon is an antioxidant as well as an antibacterial and antifungal.

MATERIALS

½ green apple, roughly chopped

2 tablespoons Greek yogurt

2 tablespoons oatmeal

½ teaspoon cinnamon

TOOLS

Blender

Facial brush

1 / Puree the green apple and yogurt together until smooth.

2 / Add the oatmeal and give the mixture a couple of pulses. You want to break down the oatmeal, but not puree it.

3 / Transfer to a clean bowl and stir in the cinnamon.

4 / Apply mask to your face with clean hands or a facial brush. Avoid the eye area.

5 / Let sit for 15 minutes and remove with warm water. Pat dry and follow with moisturizer.

TIP

What's your favorite yogurt flavor? Peach? Blueberry? Chances are it would make an awesome face mask too! The next time you reach for your breakfast yogurt, consider its versatility.

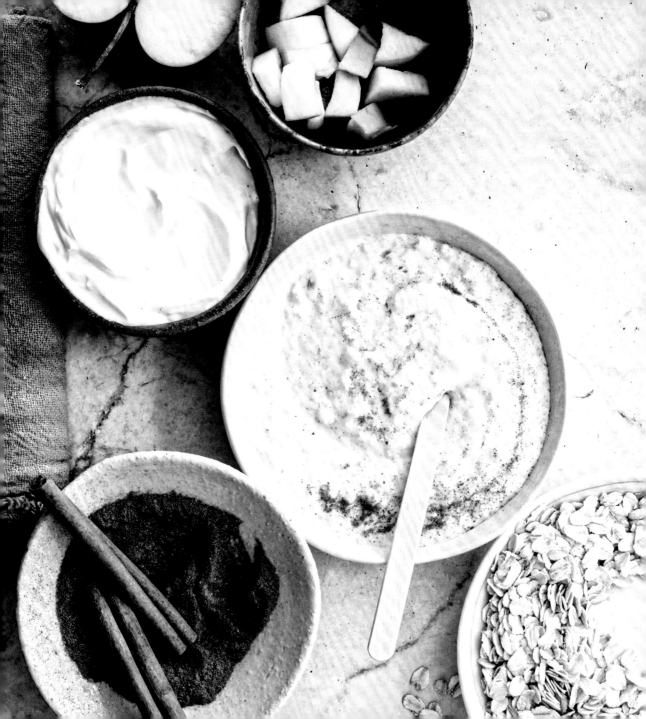

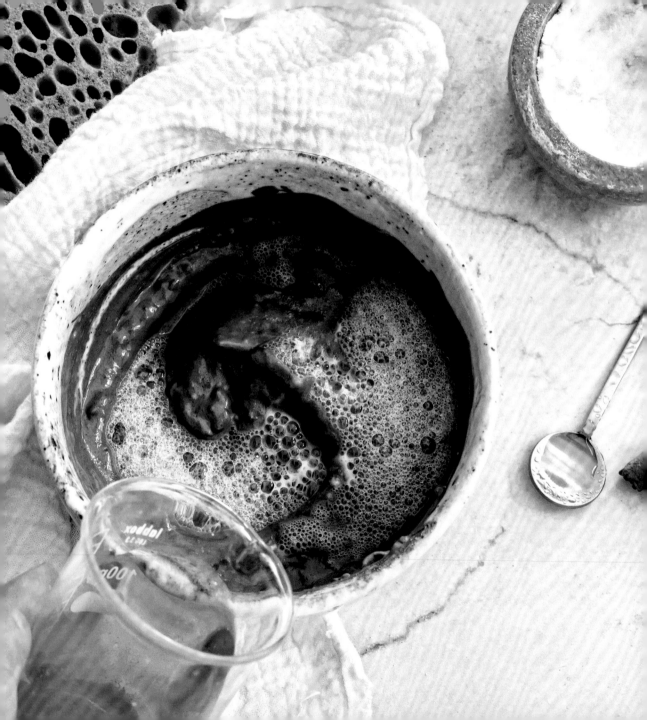

Carbonated Clay Mask

Carbonated clay masks have been a huge beauty trend, of late—and you can make your own without the cost. Instead of carbonic acid, this DIY carbonated bubble mask uses citric acid to get the same fizzy tingle.

MATERIALS

2 tablespoons rosewater

2 tablespoons bentonite clay

1 teaspoon baking soda

½ teaspoon citric acid

½ teaspoon glycerin

1 teaspoon raw honey

½ teaspoon activated charcoal or matcha powder (optional)

TIP
Not only does this homemade bubble mask massage skin, but it helps remove excess oil and tighten pores, leaving you with a fresh, clean face.

1 / Make your own rosewater using the recipe on page 53.

2 / Combine the clay, baking soda, and citric acid in a small bowl.

3 / Stir until the ingredients are well combined.

4 / For extra detox power, you can add the activated charcoal or matcha powder now too, stirring again after adding.

5 / Pour in the glycerin and honey. Stir again.

6 / At the very last minute before you use the mask, add the rosewater and stir quickly. It's going to start to fizz, so you want to work fast!

7 / Use your fingers to apply the mask to your face and neck.

8 / Let sit for 5 minutes, then use a warm washcloth to gently massage the mask into skin. Rinse your face and pat dry.

Clay + Charcoal Cleanser

Washing your face with clay and charcoal seems weird, right? But together they create a fantastic homemade facial cleanser that gently exfoliates the surface of your skin to remove makeup and dead skin cells, while also detoxifying your pores. And without the water or fresh ingredients that often cause scrubs to spoil, this cleanser will stay good for 6 months or more!

MATERIALS

¼ cup ground oats

¼ cup kaolin clay

¼ cup bentonite clay

10 capsules activated charcoal

7 drops lavender essential oil

7 drops bergamot essential oil

7 drops tea tree essential oil

TOOLS

Coffee grinder

1 / Grind oats in a coffee grinder to get a fine powder.

2 / Combine with the kaolin clay and bentonite clay in a glass mixing bowl. Be sure to measure the clay with nonmetal measuring cups.

3 / Split open the activated charcoal capsules and pour in the powder.

4 / Add the lavender, bergamot, and tea tree essential oils, and stir with a wooden spoon until well combined.

5 / Transfer to a container with a lid.

6 / To use, dispense about a teaspoon of the mixture into your hand, then add a few drops of water to create a wet paste.

7 / Gently massage into skin, making small circles with your fingers.

8 / Rinse with warm water and follow with toner and moisturizer. You can also leave the grains on your face for 10 to 15 minutes for a deep-cleansing face mask.

9 / Store in an airtight container with a lid and be careful to not introduce water.

Bentonite Clay + Chamomile Cleanser

When used regularly, gentle clay cleansers will leave skin clean, soft, exfoliated, and soothed. Personally, I love a product that can work double duty, and clay cleansers can often double as a mask with just a little extra time. This bentonite clay cleanser can work for almost any skin type—and even better, this powder cleanser can be made in a large batch and stored in a small jar for easy use.

MATERIALS

¼ cup dried calendula flowers

¼ cup dried chamomile flowers

4 tablespoons bentonite clay

1 teaspoon baking soda

½ teaspoon vitamin C powder

¼ teaspoon ground cinnamon

TOOLS

Coffee grinder

1 / Grind the dried calendula and chamomile flowers into powder using a coffee grinder.

2 / Combine the bentonite clay, baking soda, and calendula powder in a bowl.

3 / Add in the chamomile powder and vitamin C powder.

4 / Sprinkle the ground cinnamon on top, mix well, and store in a small, nonmetal jar.

5 / To use as a cleanser, shake the jar, then place a dime-sized amount (½ teaspoon) of powder in the palm of your hand, adding a few drops of water at a time until a paste is created. Rub the mixture on your face and neck for 2 minutes, then rinse and pat dry.

6 / To use as a mask, you'll want to take a little more powder so you have enough to cover your face. Mix with water, apply the mixture to your face, and leave it on for 5 to 10 minutes before rinsing thoroughly.

7 / For either use, follow with hydrating facial oil or serum.

HONEY MASKS FOR EVERY SKIN TYPE

There are some ingredients that you almost can't go wrong with when attempting DIY skincare. And honey is definitely at the top of the list. It's is naturally antibacterial, antifungal, high in antioxidants, and moisturizing. Look for raw, unfiltered honey.

FOR ACNE-PRONE SKIN

A sheet mask with chamomile tea and witch hazel calms inflammation and dries out excess oil. Honey is also anti-inflammatory and helps ward off breakouts.

¾ cup chamomile tea

¼ cup witch hazel

1 tablespoon honey

Brew tea and let it cool to room temperature. Mix in witch hazel and honey. Soak a washcloth or reusable sheet mask and apply to your skin for 15 minutes. You can store leftovers in the fridge for a week.

FOR INFLAMMATION OR SENSITIVE SKIN

Green tea and honey both work magic on redness and inflammation, making a soothing combo that is gentle enough for sensitive skin.

1 teaspoon matcha powder

1 tablespoon honey

1 teaspoon sweet almond or jojoba oil

Combine ingredients in a small bowl and mix well. (If you don't have matcha powder, cut open a green tea bag and use the leaves.) Apply to face, let sit for 15 minutes, then rinse with warm water.

SPOT TREATMENT

One-ingredient treatments are my favorite! Honey has so many uses, and fighting acne is a powerful one. Just dab honey (manuka is ideal) directly on the blemish. Leave on for 10 to 15 minutes, then rinse with warm water.

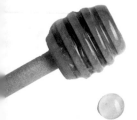

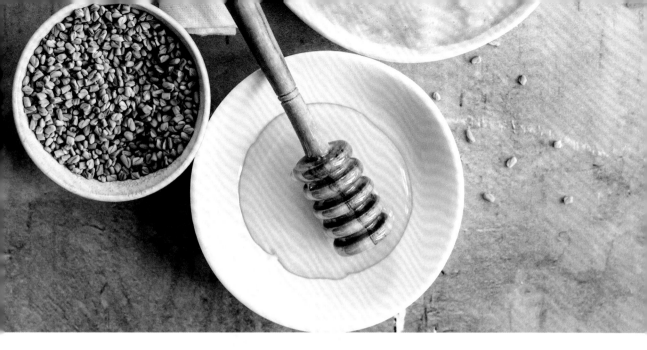

FOR DRY SKIN

With hydrating and exfoliating ingredients, plus gentle fats, this mask will leave dry skin feeling super soft. For even more moisturizing power, add a tablespoon of oil.

2 tablespoons honey

¼ avocado, mashed

2 tablespoons almonds, finely ground

Add honey and avocado to a small bowl and mash together. Stir in the ground almonds. Spread over the face and neck, and after 15 to 20 minutes, rinse with warm water.

FOR DISCOLORATION

Turmeric is used to even out skin tone and reduce the appearance of fine lines, dark spots, and scars, while lemon juice and yogurt gently exfoliate.

1 teaspoon lemon juice

1 tablespoon honey

1 tablespoon yogurt

¼ teaspoon turmeric powder

Mix all ingredients together in a small bowl. Apply in a thin layer, rest for 20 minutes, and rinse with warm water. Repeat weekly, or daily as a spot treatment. Results will take 2 to 3 months to be noticeable.

Exfoliate

Exfoliation is a crucial part of your skincare regimen, but there are so many misconceptions about how and why we exfoliate. To start with the *why*, dead skin, makeup, oil, and free radicals (another term for the yucky pollutants in our air) all take a serious toll on our skin. And that toll only grows worse as we age, and our skin self-exfoliates more slowly.

Thankfully, these masks and scrubs are here to help the skin do its job! As for the *how*, there are two types of exfoliation: natural, which uses mildly abrasive ingredients, and chemical, which uses weak acids to weaken the bonds holding dead cells in place. And lucky for you, this chapter includes both—so get ready to mix your way to better skin.

Sugar + Honey Facial Scrub

This homemade sugar scrub is formulated especially for sensitive skin. In addition to caster sugar, it's loaded with raw honey to remove debris and fight bacteria, and super-fine bentonite clay to buff away dead skin cells. In the winter, use it to remove adherent dead skin cells so moisturizers can penetrate more deeply and hydrate longer. And in summer, use it as a post-sun refresher and skin soother.

MATERIALS

1 cup caster sugar or brown sugar

¼ cup bentonite clay

1½ tablespoons grapeseed oil

1 tablespoon raw honey

15 drops Roman chamomile essential oil

½ teaspoon vitamin E oil

TIP
You only need to use this scrub about twice a week or you run the risk of overdoing it. There is a fine line between not enough exfoliation and too much exfoliation, so listen to your skin.

1 / Add the caster sugar or brown sugar and the bentonite clay to a small bowl.

2 / Pour grapeseed oil and raw honey in and stir.

3 / Finally, add the chamomile essential oil and vitamin E oil.

4 / Mix well.

5 / To use, apply a quarter-sized amount of scrub to clean skin. Using gentle circular motions, massage into skin for 60 seconds. Rinse with warm water and pat dry.

6 / If you'd like, you can store any remaining scrub in the refrigerator for up to 4 weeks.

FACIAL SCRUBS
FOR EVERY SKIN TYPE

A scrub is a great way to exfoliate, but be sure you're mixing up something gentle enough for your face, and only use it a couple times a week. You should feel glowing and fresh, but not rubbed raw! Like all exfoliation, these are best right before bed.

YOUR BASIC RECIPE

These scrubs have a mix-and-match element. Peruse your options and use:

2 tablespoons of exfoliant

2 tablespoons of oil or liquid

1 teaspoon of a skin-enhancing ingredient

Combine ingredients in a bowl and mix thoroughly. Wash face and apply scrub to damp skin with clean hands. Gently massage into your skin for about a minute, starting with the jaw and working upward, avoiding your eyes. Rinse with lukewarm water. Apply toner, then serum and moisturizer.

1 EXFOLIANTS
Start here! Depending on your skin type, choose one of the following bases.

MATURE SKIN

Ground almonds will leave mature skin nourished and hydrated while the fine grains gently exfoliate.

OILY SKIN

Baking soda not only has a super-fine texture, it also works very well at absorbing excess oil.

DRY SKIN

For a gentle exfoliation, try ground flaxseed. These seeds are hydrating, safe for acne-prone skin, and reduce wrinkles.

SENSITIVE SKIN

Oats are a good exfoliant for sensitive skin. Use them whole or grind them up.

2   LIQUID

Since this is a scrub rather than a mask, you're using less fluid—just enough to give your scrub a nice texture.

MATURE SKIN

The lactic acid in yogurt exfoliates, while the fats and proteins pump up fine lines, so go for full-fat.

OILY SKIN

Egg whites are your friend, addressing oil while also firming and tightening—bonus!

INFLAMMATION OR SENSITIVE SKIN

Aloe vera is great for keeping skin clear and healthy, on top of reducing inflammation.

DRY SKIN

Coconut oil contains fats that moisturize, while its lauric acid protects and softens skin.

3   ADD-INS

Here's where you can customize and fine-tune to get the scrub that's just right for you.

DRY SKIN

Avocado is full of good fats that moisturize dry skin. Or try raw honey, which draws in moisture.

ACNE

Turn to turmeric when you want to beat breakouts and fade acne scars.

PIGMENTATION

Pick a bit of parsley to fade age spots and treat under-eye circles.

MATURE SKIN

Avocados are rich in antioxidants—key to fighting off aging.

IRRITATION

Use raw honey on red or irritated skin to calm inflammation.

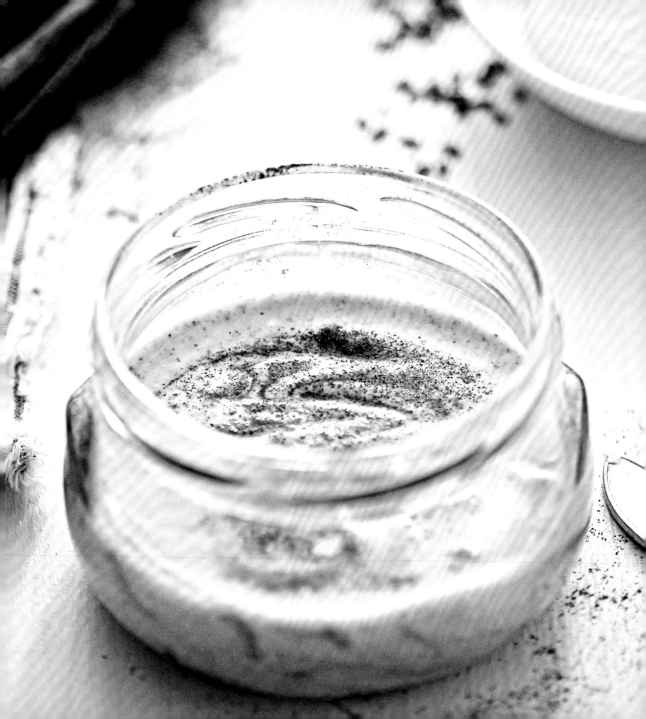

Cinnamon Flax Exfoliating Mask

This exfoliating mask is perfect for fighting acne, and absolutely fantastic for those wanting a nice, deep exfoliation. And even better, it lets you relax and pamper yourself while enjoying the wonderful smell of cinnamon.

MATERIALS

¼ cup plain yogurt

3 tablespoons ground flaxseed

1 teaspoon cinnamon

1 teaspoon honey

TOOLS

Coffee grinder

1 / Pour the yogurt into a bowl.

2 / Add the flaxseed and mix well.

3 / Sprinkle the cinnamon and honey on top.

4 / Stir until all the ingredients are evenly distributed.

5 / Apply to the face for 10 minutes before rinsing with warm water. Follow with your usual moisturizer and skincare routine.

TIP
You can buy flaxseed meal, or buy them whole and grind them up.

Grapefruit Mask

This clarifying mask is great for oily or clogged skin, and it's especially beneficial if you are battling back acne. The fruit acids will help dissolve debris and sebum in the pores, while the honey is a wonderful acne-fighting ingredient.

MATERIALS

1 tablespoon honey

½ cup cornmeal

½ grapefruit

1 / Combine honey and cornmeal in a bowl.

2 / Squeeze the juice out of the grapefruit half, letting it fall into the bowl.

3 / Mix thoroughly.

4 / Apply to your face, as well as your back, if desired.

5 / Leave on for 10 minutes and then rinse off with warm water.

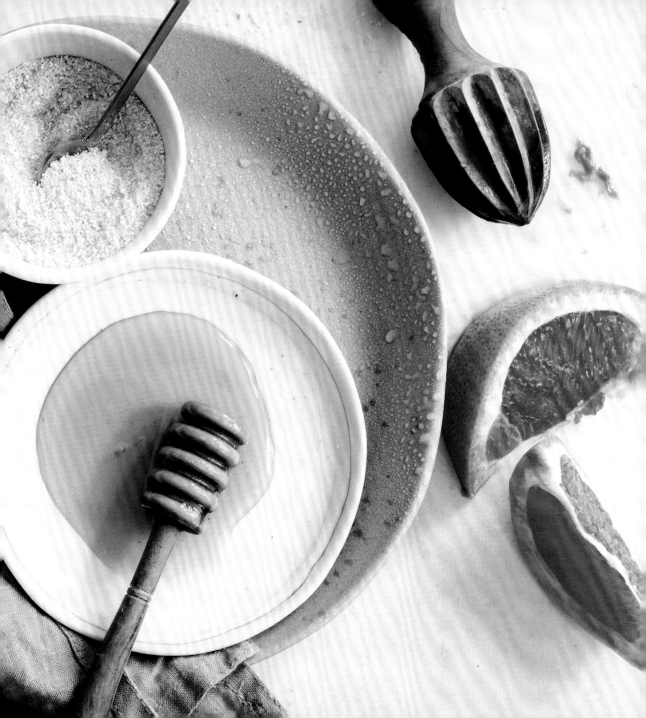

Glycolic Acid Face Mask

Glycolic acid may sound jargon-y and mysterious, but it's found in natural sources such as sugarcane, used in many different skincare products, and incredibly beneficial for your skin.

MATERIALS

2 tablespoons raw organic sugar

2 tablespoons raw honey

Juice of ½ a lemon

TOOLS

Coffee grinder or blender (optional)

1 / You'll want the sugar to be as fine as possible, so if it's coarse, you'll want to use a coffee grinder or blender to break it down.

2 / Combine the sugar and honey in a bowl.

3 / Squeeze the juice of half a lemon and mix well.

4 / Apply to the face and neck, avoiding the eye area.

5 / Rinse with warm water after just 1 to 2 minutes, and gradually increase the time before rinsing as you continue using the mask consistently, up to 5 to 10 minutes. Use this mask once a week.

Vitamin C Face Mask

Ascorbic acid, better known to us as vitamin C, plays a vital role in skin health. While taking vitamin C daily internally is known to be beneficial, applying it topically will also nourish and protect the skin. In fact, applying vitamin C to the skin gives different benefits than taking it orally—including reducing and healing damage from the sun and pollutants in the air.

MATERIALS

1 teaspoon vitamin C powder

4 teaspoons jojoba oil, or grapeseed or coconut oil

TOOLS

Facial brush

1 / In a small bowl, mix the vitamin C powder and the oil of your choosing.

2 / Blend well, until the powder is completely integrated.

3 / Apply with facial brush to face and neck.

4 / Leave on for 10 to 15 minutes and then rinse with warm water. Apply regular moisturizer and sunscreen.

5 / Feel free to apply weekly to help fight and heal damage from the environment.

TIP
Use a vitamin C powder intended for topical use—not crushed-up vitamin C that's meant to be eaten!

OATMEAL MASKS FOR EVERY SKIN TYPE

Oats are gentle, rich in antioxidants, and can help reduce inflammation, exfoliate, and cleanse the skin. You can use instant in a pinch, but never use sweetened or flavored.

MATURE SKIN 1

Super rich in vitamin C, pomegranate juice's antioxidants help fight wrinkles and dark spots while protecting the skin from free radical damage. Meanwhile, honey locks in moisture and oats calm redness and exfoliate.

1 tablespoon oats, finely ground

2 tablespoons pomegranate juice

1 teaspoon honey

Add oats to a coffee grinder and grind into a fine powder. In a bowl, combine the oats, pomegranate juice, and honey into a creamy mixture. Apply mask and relax for 15 minutes, then rinse well.

FOR DRY SKIN

This soothing mask calms inflammation and restores hydration. It can be prepared warm and will gently cool on the skin while you relax.

¼ cup warm water

¼ cup oatmeal

1 tablespoon melted coconut oil

Mix the ingredients to form a paste, and apply. Thicken or thin out the mask by changing the water content. Let sit for 10 to 15 minutes, then rinse with warm water.

FOR DULL SKIN

The natural acids in grapefruit and milk gently exfoliate and brighten skin, while oatmeal calms inflammation and soothes dry skin.

Juice from ½ ruby red grapefruit

½ cup cooked, cooled oatmeal

½ cup milk, preferably full fat

Mix ingredients in a small bowl. Apply and leave on skin for 15 minutes, then rinse.

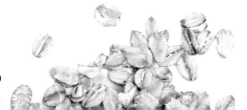

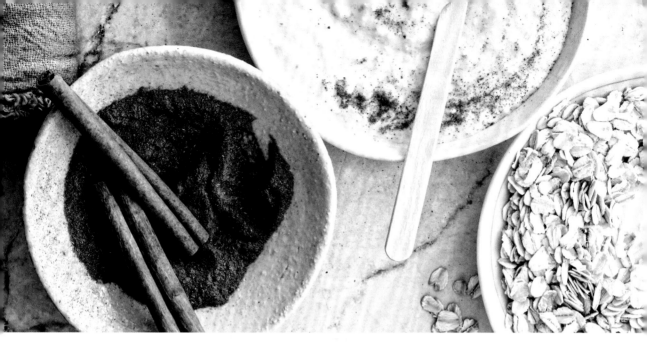

FOR GENTLE EXFOLIATION

Apple cider vinegar provides gentle exfoliation for all skin types; combined with oatmeal, it helps draw out excess oil and remove any dead cells.

1 teaspoon apple cider vinegar

¼ cup oatmeal

¼ cup warm water

Mix ingredients well in small bowl and apply to face and neck. Leave on for 5 minutes and remove with warm washcloth.

MATURE SKIN 2

Reishi mushroom is one of the most powerful mushroom adaptogens. It strengthens the skin's natural immunity, fighting radical damage and premature aging. You can find reishi mushroom in powder form, which is designed to be used in facial products, and it's generally safe for all skin types.

1 teaspoon organic reishi mushroom powder

¼ cup organic instant rolled oats

Mix reishi mushroom powder and oats in a bowl and add warm water until you achieve a paste. Leave on for 10 minutes, then remove with warm water.

Toners & Mists

Most of this book is dedicated to masks, but it would be remiss of us to leave out all of the wonderful things you can spritz on your skin! Toners and face mists fill key skincare niches, so learn how to DIY all-natural products, instead of relying on expensive, store-bought options that often contain harsh, drying alcohol.

From our Cranberry Toner to our Green Tea Face Mist, these recipes are all natural and all wonderful. Face mists not only nourish your skin, but help address dehydration and irritation—working double and triple duty. Toners, meanwhile, might seem like an afterthought, but they're also a must, especially if you're dealing with oily skin or acne. They help balance the skin's pH levels, remove stubborn traces of makeup, and prepare your skin for any additional steps in your routine. What's not to love?

Fennel + Thyme + Lemon Toner

This homemade toner is awesome for summer, when you want something light and cool on your face. I apply it straight from the fridge (via a cotton ball), and it feels heavenly. It smells pretty great, too (if you like licorice), and the soothing smell is supposed to reduce stress and tension.

MATERIALS

2 raw fennel bulbs

2 sprigs of fresh thyme

Juice of ½ a lemon

TOOLS

Blender

Cheesecloth

Covered container

Cotton balls

1 / Puree 2 bulbs of raw fennel in a blender.

2 / Add the thyme and pureed fennel to a saucepan or other small pot.

3 / Pour in enough water to make the mixture mostly liquid, ¼ to ½ cup, and bring to a boil.

4 / Once it's boiling, turn off the heat and add the lemon juice.

5 / Let steep for 15 minutes.

6 / Strain out solids with cheesecloth, transfer the remaining liquid to a covered container, and let cool.

7 / Apply to face with a cotton ball, avoiding the eyes. Do not rinse. Toner will keep in the fridge for up to 10 days; any excess can be frozen for future use.

TIP
You can also make some under-eye patches with this toner! Cut some cotton rounds (not balls) in half and soak them in the liquid, then leave them under your eyes for around 10 minutes.

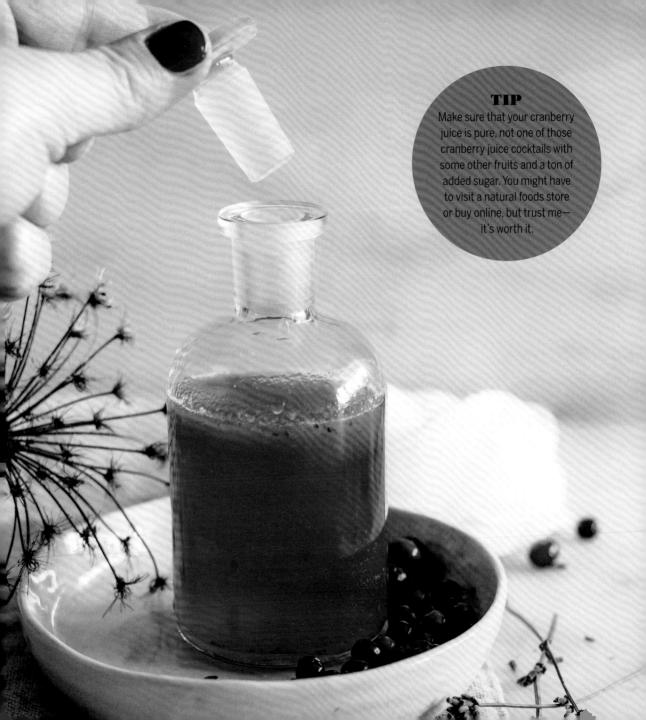

TIP

Make sure that your cranberry juice is pure, not one of those cranberry juice cocktails with some other fruits and a ton of added sugar. You might have to visit a natural foods store or buy online, but trust me—it's worth it.

Cranberry Toner

Whether you want to add a wintery-feeling twist to your skincare routine, or just love the idea of a cranberry toner, this recipe will serve you well. The antioxidants and vitamins in cranberries come together to make a true treat for your skin.

MATERIALS

2 tablespoons rosewater or lavender hydrosol

½ cup witch hazel

2 tablespoons cranberry juice

TOOLS

Funnel

6-ounce (180-mL) bottle or spray bottle

1 / If you plan to use the rosewater variation of this recipe, you can make your own using the recipe on page 53.

2 / Measure out 4 ounces (115 mL) of witch hazel and pour into a bowl.

3 / Add the cranberry juice and rosewater or lavender hydrosol, then stir.

4 / Using a funnel, slowly pour the mixture into a clean 6-ounce (180-mL) bottle.

5 / Apply to the face for 10 minutes before rinsing with warm water. Follow with your usual moisturizer and skincare routine.

6 / Let the liquid absorb into your skin before applying moisturizer. Store in the refrigerator for 2 to 4 weeks.

Lemon + Witch Hazel Toner

This witch won't cast a spell on you—but in my opinion, it is pretty magical. Witch hazel is actually a medicinal shrub that's found in North America, and has been used for generations for skin and health purposes. When you buy it, though, make sure to check the ingredients list if it's not pure—some witch hazel mixes contain up to 14 percent alcohol, which isn't exactly gentle on your skin.

MATERIALS

½ cup rosewater

½ cup alcohol-free witch hazel

1 tablespoon fresh lemon juice

TOOLS

Sealed container

Cotton balls or pads

1 / Make your own rosewater with the recipe on page 53.

2 / Stir the rosewater, witch hazel, and lemon juice together.

3 / Mix thoroughly and transfer to a sealed container.

4 / Apply toner with a cotton ball after cleaning your face and removing your makeup. Follow up with a hydrating moisturizer.

5 / Store toner in fridge and use within 1 to 2 weeks.

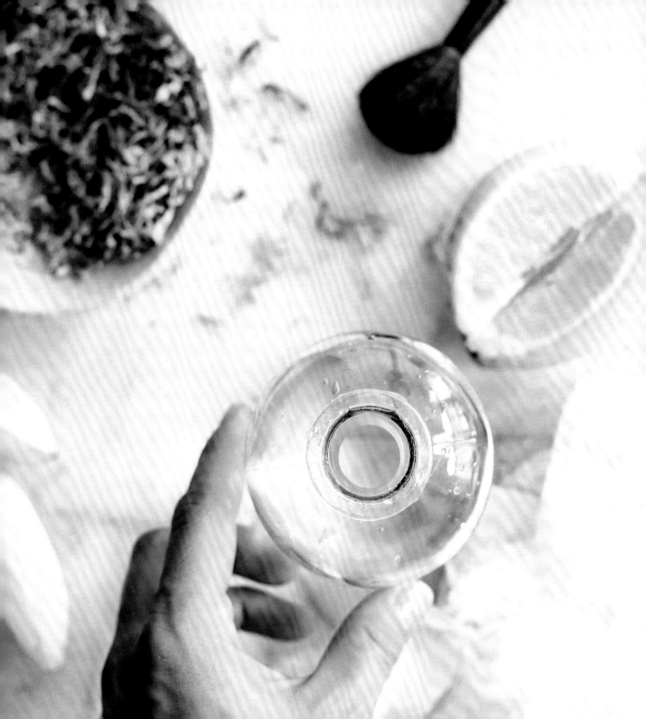

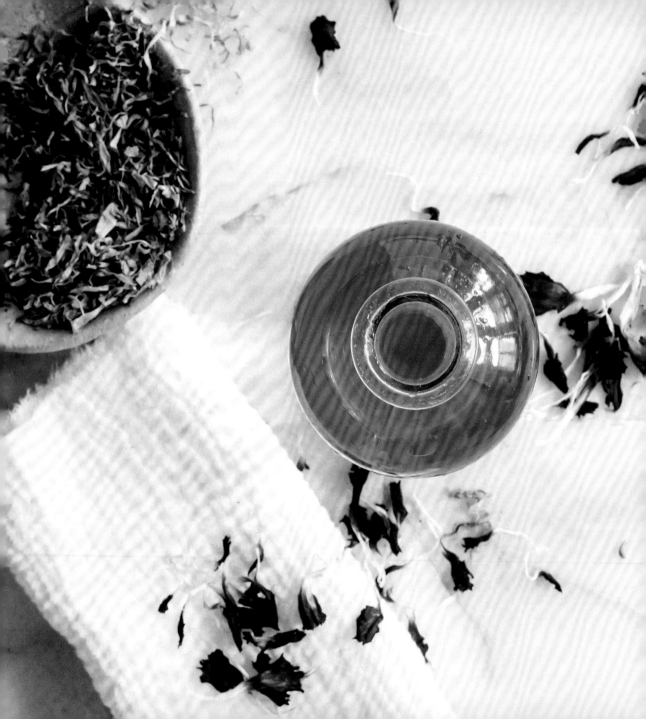

Hibiscus Tea Toner Mist

This is a simple vitamin C toner recipe that's easy to make, inexpensive, and highly effective at strengthening the skin's defenses against aging. All that, and it smells amazing too.

MATERIALS

6 ounces (180 mL) water

3 bags hibiscus tea

1 ounce (30 mL) alcohol-free witch hazel

½ teaspoon vitamin C powder

TOOLS

Small spray bottle

TIP
Start with a small amount of vitamin C powder. It breaks down quickly, losing its effectiveness, and it can also cause irritation. Work your way up to no more than 1½ teaspoons per batch of toner.

1 / Bring 6 ounces (180 mL) of water to boil.

2 / Once the water is boiling, immediately turn off heat and add three organic hibiscus tea bags.

3 / Steep covered for 20 minutes.

4 / Remove the tea bags, let the water cool to room temperature, and then add 1 ounce (30 mL) of witch hazel and ½ teaspoon of vitamin C powder.

5 / Transfer to a small spray bottle. Keep in a cool, dry spot and use within 2 weeks, or refrigerate for longer shelf life.

6 / Apply a bit to your neck to make sure you don't have any sensitivities to it, then use in the morning and at night after washing your face.

DIY Makeup Setting Spray

This makeup setting spray will help your makeup blend and stay fresh looking all day long, even out in the heat and sun. And even better, it's soothing and nourishing for dry skin.

MATERIALS

2 tablespoons rosewater

1 tablespoon filtered water

1 teaspoon aloe vera gel

½ teaspoon vegetable glycerin

2 drops frankincense essential oil

TOOLS

4-ounce (115-mL) spray bottle

Small funnel

TIP
This all-natural beauty mist is also great for soothing inflammation and irritation. While you shouldn't coat inflamed skin too heavily, a light spritz here and there can be just what your skin needs to calm the redness and promote cell turnover.

1 / Make rosewater, following the recipe on page 53.

2 / Using a funnel, pour the rosewater and filtered water into a glass spray bottle.

3 / Add the aloe vera gel and vegetable glycerin, being patient with the nonliquid ingredients if needed.

4 / Finish by dropping in the frankincense essential oil.

5 / Screw on the lid and shake thoroughly shake to combine.

6 / To apply on top of makeup,

7 / hold the bottle about twelve inches from your face and gently spritz two to three times. Allow the setting spray to dry thoroughly, without rubbing or patting it in.

8 / Store the mist in the refrigerator for up to two weeks.

Green Tea Face Mist

Tea has hydrating and refreshing effects on the skin, and makes a great base for a DIY face mist. Green tea especially is full of antioxidants and soothes irritated skin.

MATERIALS

2 organic green tea bags

1 cup hot water

4 to 6 drops argan, jojoba, or avocado oil (optional)

1 to 2 teaspoons rosewater (optional)

1 teaspoon witch hazel (optional)

TOOLS

Glass spray bottle

TIP
Store the mist in the refrigerator when you're not using it in order to preserve its potency.

1 / Steep tea bags in hot water for several minutes, then remove the tea bags.

2 / Let the tea cool to room temperature.

3 / Add any desired oils to the mist, in order to customize it to suit your skin type.

4 / Transfer tea to a glass spray bottle and shake well before each use. Simply spritz several times a day on the face and neck whenever your skin needs a refreshing boost.

Make It Your Own

Dry or Aging Skin Add 4 to 6 drops of argan, jojoba, or avocado oil to your facial mist to treat aging or dry skin—just be sure to shake well before each use. Jojoba in particular is a wonderful choice for dry skin, due to the fact that it's closely related to the oils our skin produces naturally, which makes it super easily absorbed.

Sensitive or Dry Skin Add 1 to 2 teaspoons rosewater to the mist in order to treat sensitive or dry skin. Rosewater has anti-inflammatory properties that can help out with redness and irritation.

Oily or Acne-Prone Skin Add one teaspoon of witch hazel to your green tea mist for oily or acne-prone skin. As a natural astringent, witch hazel removes excess oil on the surface of the skin, toning and soothing in the process.

51

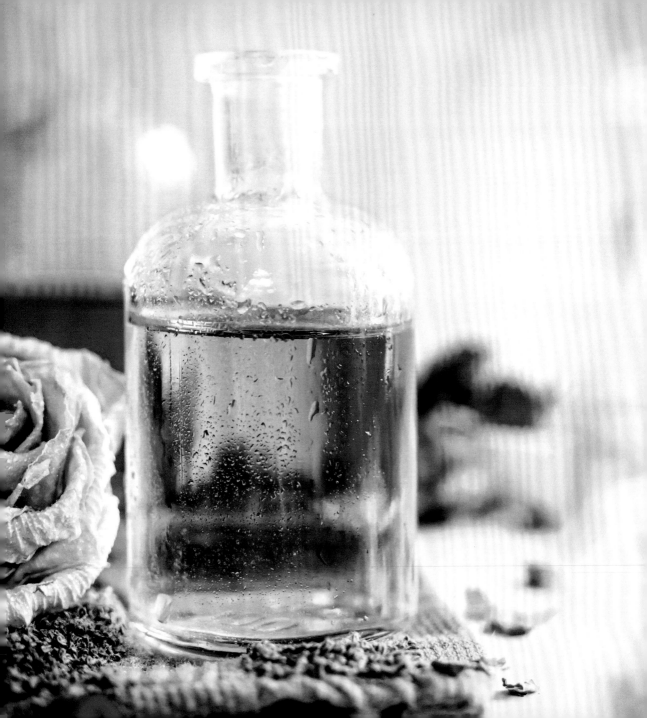

Make Your Own Rosewater

Rosewater smells delicious and makes the perfect hydrating face mist and toner. Save a few bucks and learn how to make your own! For best results, I recommend using home-grown or organic roses that are super fragrant. After all, you want to make sure you're not putting pesticides on your face!

MATERIALS

6 to 8 cups fragrant, pesticide-free rose petals

6 cups distilled water

Ice cubes

TOOLS

Heavy bowl, or cup filled with kitchen weights

Large pot with lid

Shallow, wide-mouthed bowl

Tongs

Measuring cup with spout, or kitchen funnel

Glass jar with lid, to store rosewater

1 / Remove the petals from your roses, making sure not to get any other flower parts.

2 / Place a heavy bowl or cup filled with kitchen weights in the bottom of the large pot.

3 / Then, place the shallow, wide-mouthed bowl on top of the weighted object, where it will serve as a collection bowl. Add the petals to the pot—not the bowl—spreading them around evenly. Pour 6 cups of distilled water into the pot, lightly submerging the flower petals.

4 / Place the lid on top of the pot, upside down, and pile a handful of ice cubes into the center of the upturned lid. Add more ice as needed.

5 / Simmer on medium-low for 15 to 20 minutes, until the petals begin to lose their color.

6 / Carefully remove the collection bowl from the pot with tongs, and then, using a funnel or measuring cup, pour the collected rosewater into a jar with a lid.

Eye Masks

Those three dreaded words: *you look tired.* No one wants to hear it!
But if you have dark under-eye circles or puffiness, you probably
hear it a lot. Maybe you are tired, but maybe it's genetic or your
allergies acting up. Whatever the cause, under-eye puffiness and
circles are tough to get rid of, but there are treatments for them
and if you use them consistently, those embarrassing dark spots
will fade away, leaving you looking refreshed (even if you don't
feel that way!).

    Why does the skin around the eyes always show signs of
tiredness and aging first? Well, the skin there is incredibly thin—
actually the thinnest in the body. And like any other skin issue,
prevention is more effective than treatment, so make sure you're
rested and well-hydrated, and then mix up a few of these masks.

Parsley Eye Mask

After reading that parsley can work to help erase dark eye circles, I had to try creating a recipe using it. A cure from a bunch of parsley that costs 99 cents? Really? Yep! The vitamin C, chlorophyll, and vitamin K in parsley help lighten skin discoloration, diminish age spots, and reduce puffiness.

MATERIALS

A handful of parsley, preferably organic

Yogurt (optional)

TOOLS

Cotton balls

TIP
Do this twice a week to reduce discoloration. The effects aren't immediate though; it may take several weeks to see the changes.

1 / Roughly chop a handful of parsley.

2 / In a small bowl, grind the leaves with a wooden spoon. Like muddling a drink, you want to grind the parsley until it releases the juice in the leaves.

3 / Pour a tablespoon of hot water over the parsley and stir the mixture together. You can also combine the parsley with yogurt.

4 / When the water has cooled, use 2 cotton balls to soak up the juice mixture, making sure they're well saturated.

5 / Lie down, relax, apply the cotton balls under your eyes, and rest that way for 10 minutes.

6 / You can also use as a spot treatment. Apply to any dark spots or areas of discoloration, and leave on for 10 minutes.

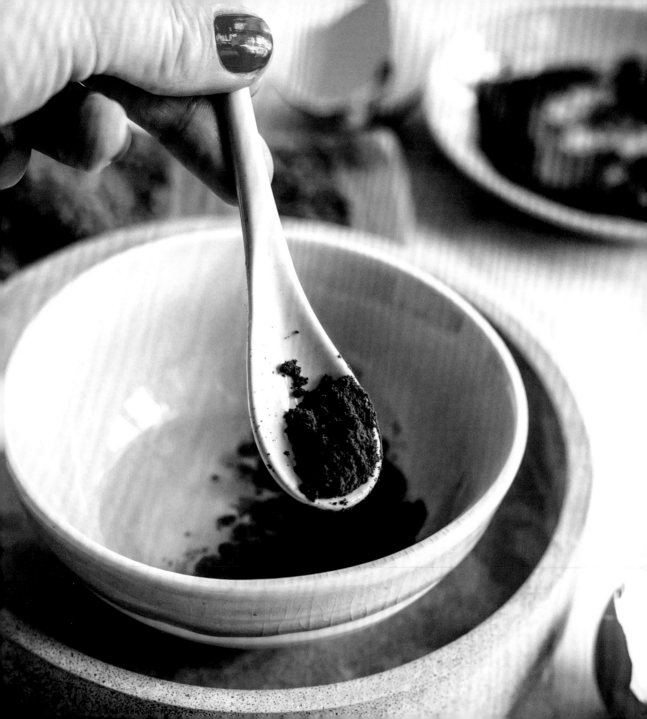

Wake-Me-Up Coffee Mask for Puffy Eyes

Erase late nights and tired eyes by adding a dose of coffee to your morning skincare routine. While you're sipping away on a cup of joe, you can also use coffee to attack dark circles and fine lines with this homemade mask for puffy eyes. And while your eyes are brighter and tighter, you may feel an internal wake-up call as the caffeine absorbs through your skin. Not bad for a 10-minute mask, right?

MATERIALS

1 egg white

2 teaspoons unused coffee grounds

1 / Combine the egg white and coffee in a small bowl.

2 / Beat the mixture together with a fork until frothy, about 1 minute.

3 / With clean hands or a brush, apply the mask around and under the eyes. You can also apply the mask to your entire face, if desired.

4 / Let the mask dry for 10 minutes. Remove with a soft, wet towel and follow with eye cream.

TIP
Unused grounds are best because they contain the most caffeine, but used grounds are fine if the coffee has just been made.

Egg White + Vitamin E Mask

You'll find egg whites in many anti-wrinkle masks for the face, and the eye area is no exception. Egg whites have been known to reduce the appearance of fine lines, while antioxidant rich vitamin E fights free radicals. The necessary vitamin E for this mask can be extracted from vitamin E capsules or found in vitamin E oil.

MATERIALS

2 egg whites

1 capsule or 5 drops of vitamin E oil

1 / Beat the egg whites with a fork until they're frothy, which will take about 1 minute.

2 / Pour into a bowl and mix in the vitamin E capsule or oil.

3 / Apply the mixture to the under-eye area with your fingertips or a makeup brush, careful not to ignore the outer edges of the eyes, where expression and squint lines form.

4 / Leave on for 10 minutes, then rinse.

Milk + Turmeric Mask

Turmeric masks are excellent for brightening complexions and evening out skin tone, and they even work on pesky dark circles. Combine with milk for a bit of gentle exfoliation.

MATERIALS

1 teaspoon turmeric

1 tablespoon milk or buttermilk

TOOLS

Facial brush

1 / Mix the turmeric and milk (or buttermilk) together in a small bowl until thoroughly blended.

2 / Use a brush to paint the mask onto your under-eye area, avoiding the eyes.

3 / Leave on for 15 minutes and then carefully wipe off the mask. Follow with moisturizer.

Cucumber + Rose Eye Mask

Ever wonder why sliced cucumbers are always shown in spa scenes on TV? It's because they're so incredibly effective. Rich in ascorbic acid and phytochemicals, cucumbers help tighten and soothe skin. But unlike simple cucumber slices, this blended mask will reach the inner and outer corners of your eyes with concentrated vitamins and minerals.

MATERIALS

1 ounce (30 mL) rosewater

½ cucumber

TOOLS

Cotton rounds

Blender

1 / Make your own rosewater with the recipe on page 53.

2 / Cut your cotton rounds into half-moon shapes. This mask makes a lot, so cut more than you think you'll need.

3 / In a blender, puree the cucumber and rosewater until liquified.

4 / Transfer to a bowl, then soak the cotton rounds in the mixture, squeezing out excess and then resoaking for optimal absorption.

5 / Store the extra soaked cotton rounds in a Ziploc bag in the freezer for future use.

6 / Thaw the eye pads for about 10 minutes before you use them, but make sure they are still cool, as the temperature will also help with reducing puffiness.

7 / To apply, place the half-moon eye pad underneath the eye, making sure to apply close to the bottom lash line. Leave on for 10 to 15 minutes.

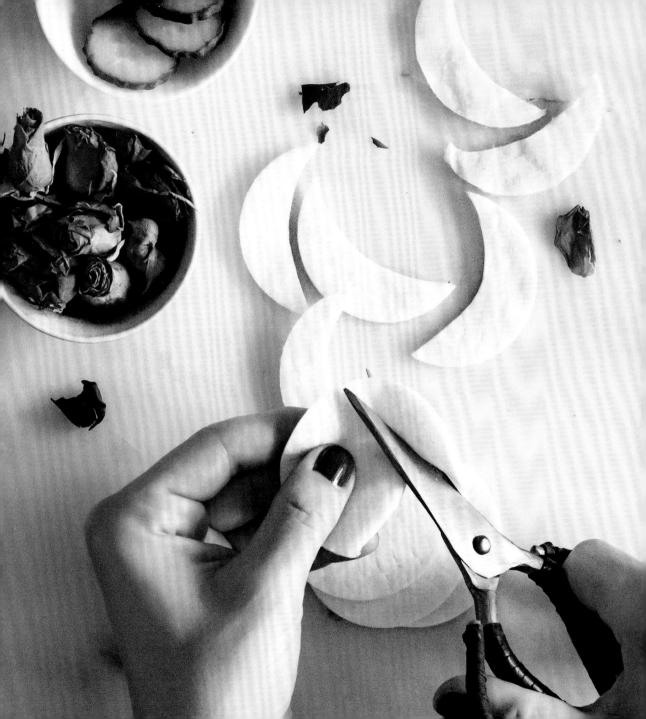

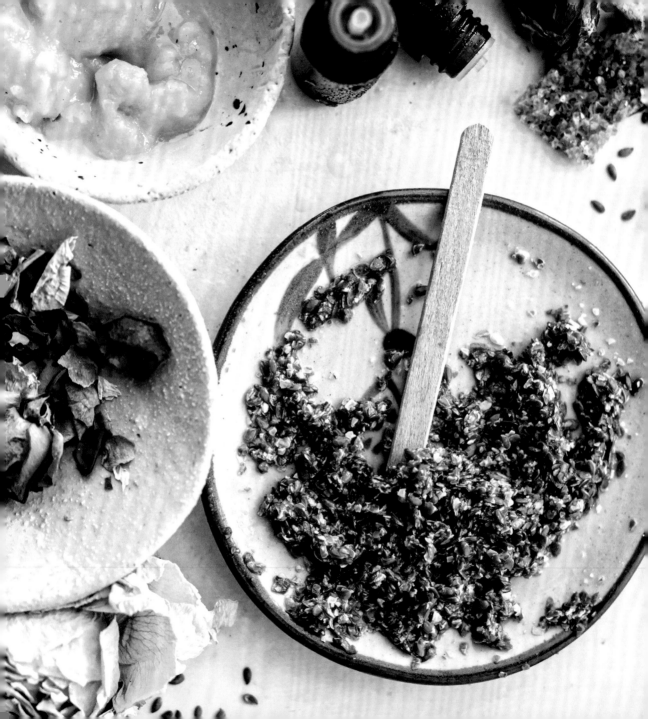

Flaxseed Gel Eye Mask

Flaxseed is a superfood you might not have heard of, but that you should look into using immediately. Not only are the seeds nutritious, they provide massive beauty benefits when applied directly to the skin, helping to nourish skin, balance oil, and provide nutrients. And a flaxseed gel eye mask like the one below is great at softening fine lines and wrinkles.

MATERIALS

1 tablespoon rosewater

3 tablespoons filtered water

½ teaspoon raw honey

2 drops Roman chamomile essential oil

2 tablespoons flaxseed

TIP
Flaxseed is also great for putting in your body, not just on it! Try adding ground flaxseed to salad dressings or smoothies, yogurt or oatmeal, or any baked goods you're preparing.

1 / Make your own rosewater with the recipe on page 53.

2 / Pour the filtered water and rosewater into a bowl.

3 / Add the honey and chamomile essential oil, stirring thoroughly to ensure they're spread throughout the mixture.

4 / Mix in flaxseed and stir well.

5 / Allow the mixture to soak for about 10 minutes. Over time, the flaxseed will form a somewhat thick, gel-like substance—that's the mask.

6 / If you find that the gel has thickened a little too much, add a teaspoon of filtered water to thin it just enough to spread evenly over your skin.

7 / Apply the gel to under-eye skin and let sit for 15 to 20 minutes.

8 / To remove, moisten mask with water and massage mask into your skin for 2 minutes.

9 / Rinse with lukewarm water. Throw away any unused mask.

Lip Masks

We tend to think more about lip care in winter when we're applying lip balm 20 times a day to handle super dry, chapped lips. But that doesn't mean that our lips are free of issues after a crisp autumn breeze, a cross-country flight, or a relaxing day at the beach. Your lips get a workout every day just with smiling, talking and eating, and yet the delicate skin has no sebum-producing glands to help it stay moist and protected—hence the size of your Chapstick budget.

So it's lucky, then, that masks and scrubs aren't just for your face. Give your lips a turn being pampered, and mix up these healing, exfoliating, and plumping recipes. Trust me—your lips will thank you.

Plumping Lip Mask

Celebs are often spotted on Instagram using collagen-infused lip masks to plump their lips. You can get the same effect at home with a couple of mega-moisturizing ingredients.

Sunflower and safflower oil both contain linoleic acid, an essential fatty acid that moisturizes, restores, and plumps up the uppermost layer of skin on your lips. And raw honey acts as a humectant to draw in moisture, on top of its antibacterial and anti-inflammatory properties.

MATERIALS

1 teaspoon sunflower oil or safflower oil

1 tablespoon honey

TOOLS

Plastic wrap

1 / Pour the sunflower or safflower oil into a bowl.

2 / Add in the honey and mix thoroughly.

3 / Apply all over and around the lips.

4 / Cover with a small piece of plastic wrap, which will help lock in the heat and intensify the mask's effectiveness.

5 / Leave on for 5 minutes, then wash off using warm water.

TIP
If you want to add in some exfoliation power, add a pinch of brown sugar to the oil and honey mixture. Then massage gently into the lips to loosen any dead, dry skin.

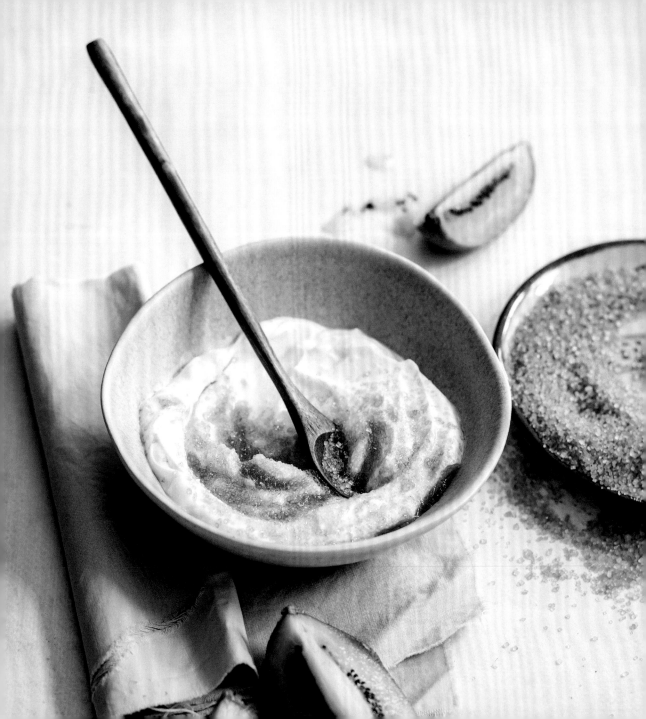

Exfoliating Kiwi Lip Mask

If your lips are tender, exfoliating with a scrub can hurt. Which is why this lip peel uses the natural alpha hydroxy acids in yogurt (lactic acid), cane sugar (glycolic acid), and kiwi (citric acid) to get rid of dead skin instead.

The acids help break down the bonds that hold our dead skin cells together, releasing them without any manual scrubbing. Think of this mask as a kind of peel, because the exfoliation is more chemical than physical. But it's still gentle, don't worry!

MATERIALS

1 teaspoon Greek yogurt

¼ teaspoon cane sugar

1 slice kiwi, about ½ to 1 teaspoon

TOOLS

Plastic wrap

1 / Combine the yogurt and sugar in a bowl.

2 / Let the mixture sit for a few minutes so that the sugar dissolves into the yogurt.

3 / Then mash in a bit of kiwi and stir.

4 / Apply the mask all over your lips, then cover them with a small piece of plastic wrap.

5 / Let sit for 5 minutes and then rinse with warm water.

Rose
Compress

My chapped lips loved this soothing mixture, which uses milk's lactic acid to exfoliate, and is much gentler than using a scrub. Rose oil is anti-inflammatory, to ease irritated skin, and the subtle rose smell and flavor is a relaxing bonus.

MATERIALS

2 tablespoons milk

1 drop rose absolute essential oil

TOOLS

Cotton balls

1 / Combine the milk and rose essential oil in a small dish.

2 / Stir well.

3 / Dip a cotton ball into the mixture and apply to the lips.

4 / Let the liquid sit on your lips for 5 minutes—you can hold the cotton ball to your lips if you want.

5 / Refrigerate any extra and use within 2 weeks.

Lavender Latte Lip Scrub

Coffee grounds buff away dry skin, while honey is a humectant to attract and lock in moisture. Top it all off by adding a drop of healing lavender oil to soothe irritated skin.

MATERIALS

1 tablespoon ground coffee

½ to 1 tablespoon honey

1 drop lavender essential oil

1 / In a small bowl, combine the coffee grounds and honey.

2 / Add the lavender essential oil and mix well.

3 / Smooth a small amount of the scrub onto clean, dry lips.

4 / Let the mixture sit on your lips for 30 seconds, and then massage your lips with a fingertip.

5 / Rinse and follow with lip balm. You can store any extra mixture in a small jar in the fridge.

TIP
It's best to use full coffee grounds so they retain their full potency, but using grounds from very freshly brewed coffee also works.

Serums

As time goes on, it seems like there's an ever-growing number of skincare products we have to use. Everyone knows about cleansers, and then there's moisturizing, and then there's so many, many different things—including serums. But being one product of many doesn't mean that facial serums aren't important. They are, I promise. Facial serums are typically an oil- or water-based treatment that delivers highly concentrated, targeted nutrients to address one or more skin problems. That makes serums an important tool in your skincare toolkit.

Good serums can be pricey, though—which is why you should try out the following homemade options. DIYing serums has so many benefits: It's less expensive, totally customizable for your own skin, and as easy as mixing a few oils together.

Acne-Fighting Chamomile Face Serum

Chamomile essential oil will calm irritated and inflamed skin, while aloe is anti-inflammatory and hydrating, boosting your skin's natural healing abilities. Lavender, tea tree, and frankincense essential oils are all effective at diminishing acne and scarring, and can be swapped out for the chamomile oil if you don't already have it on hand.

MATERIALS

Roman chamomile essential oil, 2 drops per 1 ounce (30 mL) of carrier oil

Grapeseed, hemp, or jojoba oil to serve as a carrier oil

Aloe vera gel

TOOLS

Dark glass bottle

1 / Mix the Roman chamomile essential oil into your chosen carrier oil using 2 essential oil drops per 1 ounce (30 mL) of carrier oil.

2 / Store the oil mixture in a dark glass bottle, but do *not* add the aloe vera.

3 / Add the aloe vera gel to the serum right before each use in order to avoid spoilage.

4 / To use, place a pea-sized amount of the oil in the palm of your hand and add a few drops of aloe vera gel. Mix together, then apply all over your face and neck.

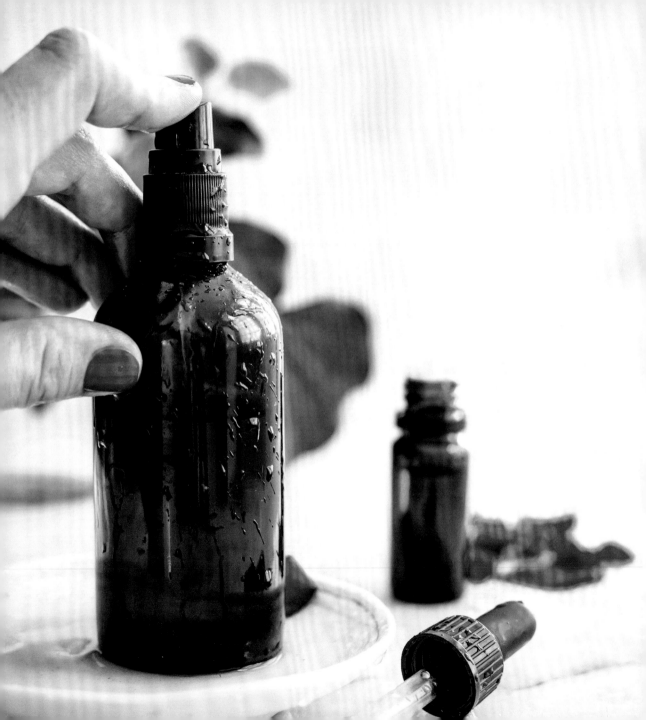

Rosehip + Rosewater Face Serum

Since this oil is oh so fabulous, I wanted to use it to make a serum that not only does amazing things for your skin, but smells amazing as well. Luckily, all it requires is mixing up a few simple ingredients that you probably already have.

MATERIALS

1 tablespoon rosewater

25 to 30 drops rosehip seed oil

1 tablespoon avocado, almond, or jojoba oil

3 drops geranium essential oil (optional)

3 drops ylang ylang essential oil (optional)

TOOLS

2-ounce (60-mL) spray bottle or roll-on applicator

1 / Make your own rosewater using the recipe on page 53.

2 / Combine the rosewater and rosehip seed oil in the bottle.

3 / Add in your choice of the avocado, almond, or jojoba oil.

4 / Shake well to combine.

5 / If the mixture isn't fragrant enough for you, add more rosewater—or even a few drops of geranium or ylang ylang essential oils. That's the beauty of DIY: tailoring any recipe to suit you.

6 / Shake well before each use, and apply this super moisturizing serum on your face at night after cleansing and first thing in the morning.

NOTE You can also put the serum in a mister bottle and mist throughout the day to alleviate dry skin. Keep the mister bottle in the fridge, especially in the summer! This does two really important things—first, how good does a cold spray feel on a hot summer day? Amazing, right? Second, keeping this solution cold ensures that it stays fresher for longer—and at its most potent.

Hydrating Jojoba + Frankincense Face Serum

At night, I still slather on face oil. But for daytime, I've switched to a lighter aloe vera and carrier oil serum. It feels light and smooth—perfect for wearing under a daytime natural makeup look. I love aloe vera—we need more beauty ingredients that multitask as much as we do!

MATERIALS

1 tablespoon aloe vera gel

1 tablespoon jojoba oil

6 drops frankincense essential oil

TOOLS

Funnel

Small bottle with dropper lid

1 / Use a funnel to pour the aloe vera into a small bottle with a dropper lid.

2 / Still using the funnel, pour in the jojoba oil and frankincense essential oil.

3 / Put the lid on the bottle and shake until the ingredients are all mixed thoroughly.

4 / Shake the bottle well before each use and apply the serum to a clean, damp face.

Pomegranate Face Serum

This wonderful serum calms almost any dry, itchy skin condition. Pomegranate seed oil deeply penetrates the skin to improve skin healing. Avocado oil is loaded with vitamins A and D, as well as fatty acids that improve skin hydration and elasticity. And rosehip seed oil, my favorite, has lots of vitamin C and natural retinol to help reverse sun damage.

MATERIALS

2 teaspoons avocado oil

2 teaspoons pomegranate seed oil

2 teaspoons rosehip seed oil

3 drops frankincense essential oil

3 drops Roman chamomile or lavender essential oil

TOOLS

Small bottle with dropper lid

1 / Add the avocado, pomegranate, and rosehip seed oils to the bottle.

2 / Add essential oils and swirl.

3 / Screw on the lid cover and shake the bottle to thoroughly mix ingredients.

4 / Apply 2 to 4 drops to your fingers and pat onto your face. Don't rub or pull the skin.

TIP
This serum is especially great for the winter months, given the damage the cold and wind all too often do to skin.

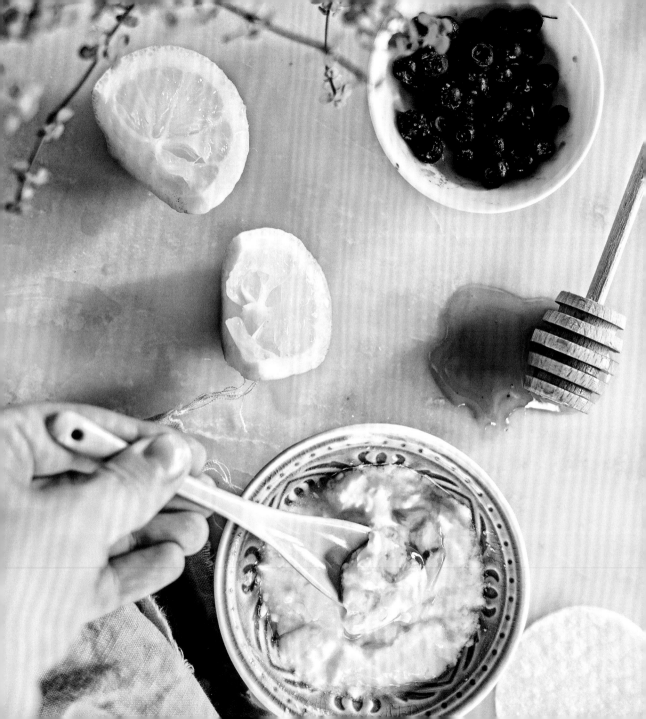

Part 2
Personalize Your Skincare Routine

Soothe & Nurture

We live in a world that is all too often not kind to our skin—unfortunately. But when things get irritated, inflamed, or sensitive, these masks can come to the rescue. Think of these masks as dedicated TLC for irritation, as well as nourishing care for skin that's doing well—because there's no such thing as too much pampering. But if your skin is telling you that something is wrong, these masks are the perfect tools to calm it down.

Some of these masks are great for sensitive skin specifically, but all skin experiences bad days or weeks or months. Maybe there's been too much winter dryness, maybe it's been exposed to too many irritants. Whatever the case, these masks can help you soothe your skin and return it to a gorgeous, glowing health.

Overnight Oat Milk Mask

Because they're chock full of things like phenols, saponins, and beta-glucans, oats are said to help soothe inflammation while also cleansing and hydrating the skin. We don't recommend leaving oats on your face all night (that can get ugly, fast), but you can reap many of the same benefits from oat milk—without the mess.

MATERIALS

2 tablespoons organic oat milk

½ teaspoon raw honey

1 drop lavender essential oil

1 drop chamomile essential oil

TOOLS

Cotton balls

1 / Mix together oat milk and raw honey into a small bowl.

2 / Add in the lavender and chamomile essential oils, stirring thoroughly.

3 / Apply to your face using a cotton ball and let it dry a bit before you hit the hay. Rinse with cool water in the morning.

TIP
This mask is best for oily skin. If you have dry skin, skip it entirely or apply it only to your T-zone.

Pumpkin Bread Foodie Face Mask

I'm sure I'm not the only one with a true love for sweater weather—and pumpkin-flavored everything. But pumpkin isn't just a fall favorite! It's is packed with vitamins, minerals, and enzymes that help moisturize dry skin, repair sun damage, maintain healthy oil production, and encourage cell turnover. And that's before all the benefits of these additional ingredients. Also, this mask smells like a fresh loaf of pumpkin bread. Can't forget that benefit!

MATERIALS

¼ cup pumpkin puree

½ teaspoon ground cinnamon

¼ teaspoon ground nutmeg

¼ teaspoon ground ginger

1 tablespoon finely ground almond meal

TOOLS

Blender

1 / Puree ¼ cup pumpkin meat in a blender, making sure to remove all the seeds. (If you don't want to make your own pumpkin puree, store bought is fine.)

2 / Plop the pumpkin puree into a bowl, add the cinnamon, nutmeg, and ginger, and stir.

3 / Stir in the almond meal.

4 / Mix until the mask has attained a lovely, even texture.

5 / Apply the mask to a freshly washed face (and neck, if you like) with your fingers, spreading it on with a gentle, circular motion.

6 / Sit back and relax as you let the ingredients work their magic for 15 to 20 minutes.

7 / Wash the mask off with warm water and a soft washcloth, then apply your usual moisturizer.

8 / Store any remaining mask in the fridge and use within a few days.

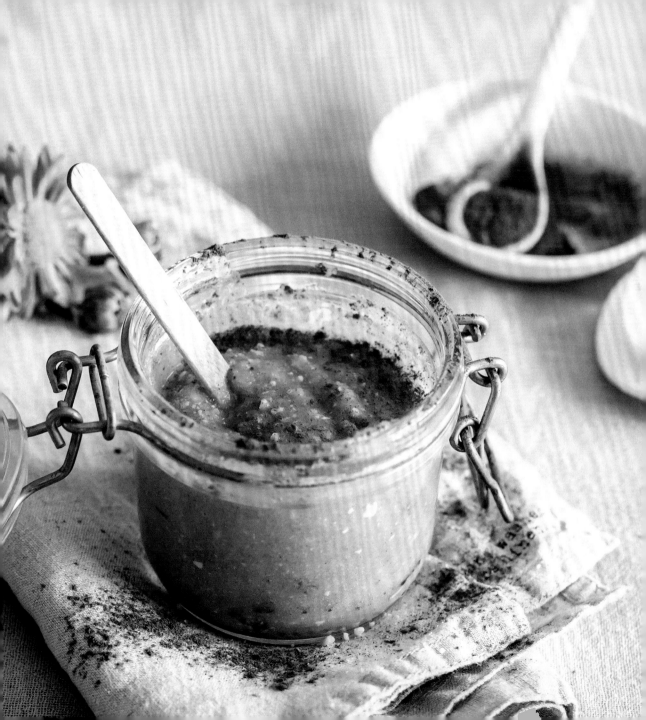

Seaweed Sheet Mask

Seaweed's natural anti-inflammatory and exfoliant properties make it a perfect choice for those suffering from acne or rosacea. The vitamins found in seaweed can help ease the swelling and redness often associated with breakouts, and lessen the pooling of blood beneath the skin for those with rosacea.

MATERIALS

Filtered water or green tea

A few sheets of organic nori seaweed

1 / Place filtered water—or green tea, if you want to focus on the mask's anti-aging benefits—in a plate that has a small lip so nothing spills over.

2 / Dip the seaweed in the water for just a second or two, so it's quickly moistened.

3 / Tear the sheets into smaller pieces for the areas around your nose and mouth if you'd like.

4 / Place the moistened sheets all over your face—you'll need about 3 to 5 sheets depending on the size of the seaweed, and several more if you are including your neck.

5 / Leave the sheet mask on for 10 to 15 minutes and then peel off, rinse, and follow with a moisturizer.

Soothing Agar Peel Off

What is agar and how can we use it? Agar (or agar-agar) is made from seaweed—more specifically red algae. It softens and moisturizes skin; it also helps thicken and bind other ingredients together. This mask, while hydrating, is also a great exfoliating mask, removing surface dead skin cells as you peel it off, revealing glowing and fresh skin.

MATERIALS

2 tablespoons milk

1 tablespoon agar powder

1 teaspoon honey

2 drops chamomile essential oil or tea tree oil

1 capsule vitamin E oil (optional)

NOTE

While applying the mask, be sure to avoid the eyebrows and the eye area, as it can pull and tug during removal. Apply an even layer—a clean, flat makeup brush is helpful here—concentrating on any area with clogged pores or blackheads. And if you need help removing it, use a bit of warm water—don't try to force it!

1 / Steam milk in a heat-safe bowl.

2 / Before it cools, add the agar powder and mix well.

3 / Pour in the honey and chamomile essential oil (or tea tree oil, if you have acne-prone skin), and keep mixing until the consistency is even.

4 / Break open a vitamin E capsule and stir in, if desired. This will make the mask better for dry or aging skin.

5 / Apply, avoiding the eye area, while the mask is still warm, but not hot. If you're not sure, dab a little on the inside of your wrist. The mask should be comfortably warm on your face. If you put it on and it's a little too hot, rinse it off right away to avoid burns.

6 / Once the mask is dry—usually 10 to 20 minutes—you'll feel your face tighten. Start to peel in an upward motion, beginning with the chin area and going all the way to the forehead. The mask may peel off in several sections, which is fine.

7 / After you've peeled off most of it, use a warm washcloth and remove any leftover mask. Finish with a hydrating moisturizer or serum.

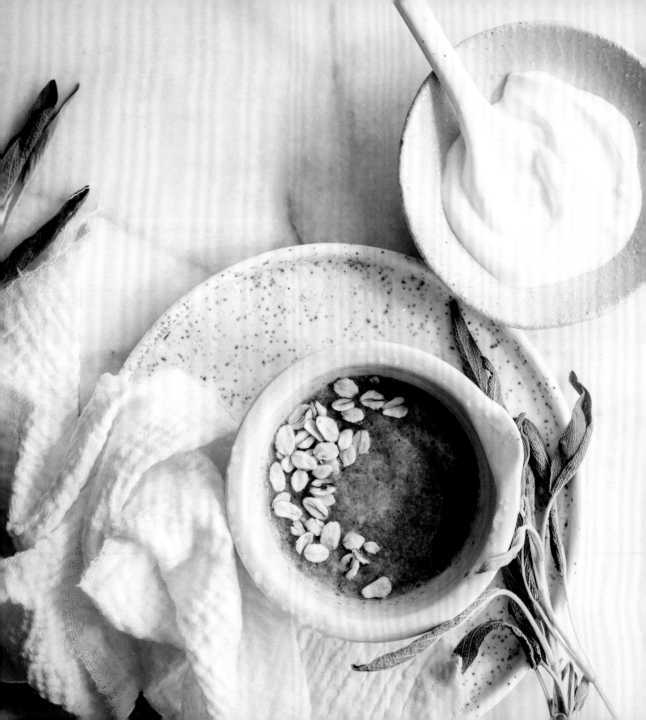

Calming Cucumber Mask

Winter air can leave skin dry and parched—but this calming and hydrating face mask will take the red right out of those windburned cheeks. Cucumber and oatmeal are both anti-inflammatory, sage is an antioxidant, and yogurt is one of the simplest and most effective face mask ingredients because it soothes and gently exfoliates.

MATERIALS

2 tablespoons pureed cucumber

2 tablespoons plain yogurt

2 tablespoons oats, uncooked

1 teaspoon chopped, fresh sage

TOOLS

Blender

1 / Puree a whole cucumber in a blender and measure out 2 tablespoons of ingredient.

2 / Add the cucumber to a bowl, and follow with yogurt, oatmeal, and finely chopped sage.

3 / Mix ingredients thoroughly. Note that the sage and oatmeal mean the texture of the mask will not be smooth, but they should still be evenly spread throughout.

4 / Massage the finished mask into clean, damp skin.

5 / Relax with this mask on for 15 minutes, then rinse to remove.

YOGURT MASKS FOR EVERY SKIN TYPE

Sometimes the best ingredients for your skin are the easiest to find. Plain, preservative-free yogurt contains lactic acid that gently dissolves dead skin cells, unclogs pores, and evens skin tone.

SENSITIVE SKIN REFRESHER

For reactive skin, keep it simple. Using just plain yogurt with live cultures and no preservatives, apply a thin layer to the face and neck, and leave on for 15 to 20 minutes. Rinse with warm water.

FOR MATURE SKIN 1

A mix of berries is a great way to get an all-around effective mask. Strawberries are rich in vitamin C and folate, while blackberries contain potent antioxidants.

2 tablespoons plain yogurt

¼ cup mixed berries

Combine in a blender and pulse until smooth. Apply and leave on for 10 to 20 minutes before rinsing.

FOR MATURE SKIN 2

Combine yogurt's natural probiotics and gentle exfoliation with vitamin-rich pumpkin to help even out skin tone, clean pores, and fade age spots.

1 tablespoon canned pumpkin

1 tablespoon Greek yogurt

Mix ingredients together and apply to a clean face. Let the mask do its magic for 15 minutes, then rinse with warm water.

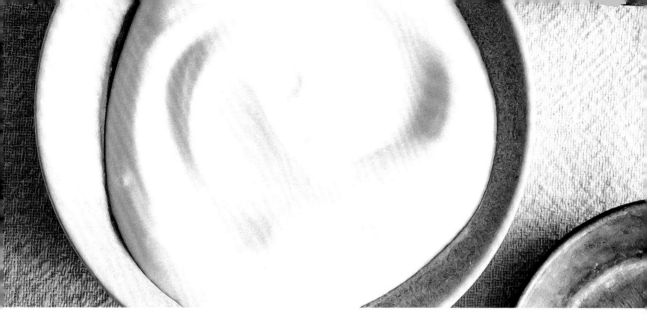

FOR DRY SKIN

Say goodbye to dry skin with this mask-meets-scrub treatment that nourishes and hydrates while it whisks away dead skin cells.

**¼ cup cooked carrots, cooled
(you can also use baby food)**

2 tablespoons yogurt

1 tablespoon white sugar

Blend the carrots with the yogurt, then stir in the sugar. Gently massage into the skin for 2 minutes, then relax and let the mask sit for 15 minutes. Rinse with warm water.

FOR DULL SKIN

Blueberries and lemon are incredibly rich in vitamin C, which appears in a lot of commercial serums designed to brighten dull skin and even out skin tone. Meanwhile, honey draws moisture into the skin for a radiant boost.

2 tablespoons of plain organic yogurt

1 to 2 teaspoons honey

A squeeze of lemon juice

Small handful of blueberries, preferably organic

Blend ingredients together until you get a creamy paste, then liberally apply to your face and neck. Leave the mask on for 20 minutes, then wash off with warm water.

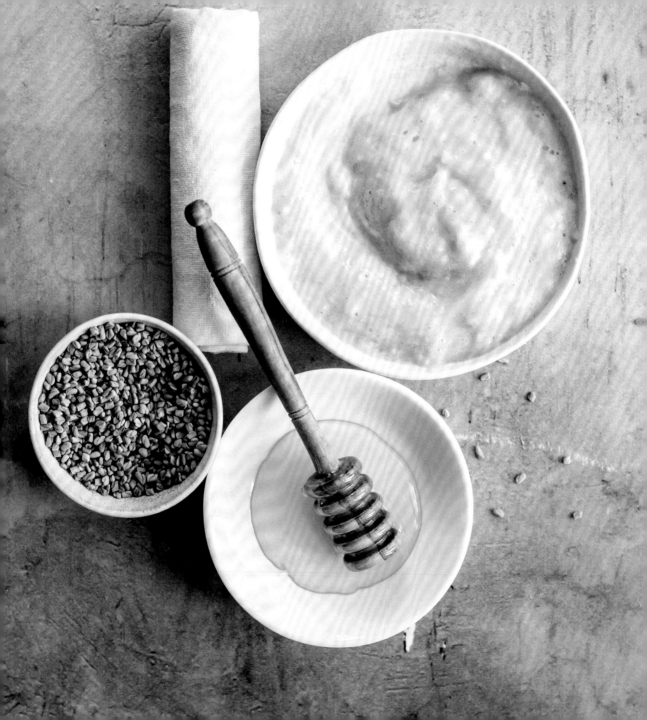

Simple Fenugreek Seed Face Mask

Fenugreek seeds might be in your spice rack right now, but did you know they have multiple uses beyond the kitchen? And one of the best ways to use them is to whip up a fenugreek seed face mask. These healing seeds can be used for every skin type, and are praised for their anti-inflammatory and antioxidant abilities. And even better, you don't need to add a long grocery list of ingredients to them in order to reap their benefits. They're super potent on their own.

MATERIALS

1 cup fenugreek seeds

2 cups water

1 teaspoon honey

TOOLS

Blender

1 / In a covered bowl, soak the fenugreek seeds in water overnight.

2 / The next day, add only the seeds and honey to a blender and blend until a paste forms. Set aside the water that the seeds soaked in for later.

3 / Apply to face and neck and leave on for 20 minutes. It will be thick, but don't worry—it's supposed to be!

4 / Rinse with lukewarm water. Follow with moisturizer to lock in that glow!

Help Out Your Hair

What about that fenugreek water that we put aside? Well, that's perfect for using on your hair. Put the leftover liquid into a spritz bottle and spray liberally over your scalp and hair, mainly focusing on the roots but still getting it on the length of your hair. You can leave it on for the same amount of time as your mask (just rinse out after!), or for a super intensive treatment, you can leave it on overnight. After washing it out of your hair, your locks will look super shiny and luscious—I promise!

Matcha Green Tea Mask

Green tea is all-round awesome. It is seriously one of the best things to put on your face in summer. Its fancy-pants polyphenols help protect the skin from the sun, while the catechins go forth and fight aging and sun damage. There's just a lot to love. On top of that, honey soothes and cinnamon stimulates blood flow, while sandalwood essential oil nourishes, making this combination a wonderful skin rejuvenator.

MATERIALS

½ tablespoon boiled water

1 tablespoon matcha green tea powder

1 teaspoon honey

1 drop of sandalwood essential oil

A pinch cinnamon (optional, not for sensitive skin)

1 / Set water to boil in preparation for later use.

2 / Pour the honey and matcha powder into a bowl.

3 / Add the sandalwood essential oil, and a pinch of cinnamon if desired.

4 / Mix thoroughly, while adding the water slowly, until you reach a consistency thick enough to apply.

5 / Apply to face (avoiding the eye area) and neck.

6 / Relax for 20 minutes, then rinse off, tone, and moisturize.

Cactus Water Mask

The idea of putting anything cactus related on your face might sound a bit, well, scary. Especially something derived from a plant called "prickly pear." But the pretty, pink water sourced from the fruit of said cactus is actually packed with antioxidants that nourish and hydrate the skin, inside and out.

MATERIALS

1 ounce (30 mL) cactus water

1 ounce (30 mL) aloe vera

¼ teaspoon vitamin C powder

1 tablespoon pink clay

1 teaspoon prickly pear seed oil, or ½ teaspoon prickly pear and ½ teaspoon jojoba oil

1 drop rose essential oil

2 drops frankincense essential oil

2 drops helichrysum essential oil

TOOLS

Facial brush (optional)

1 / In a measuring cup or small bowl, combine the cactus water and aloe vera.

2 / Add vitamin C powder and stir until dissolved.

3 / Add pink clay and stir until combined.

4 / In a separate bowl, combine prickly pear seed oil or prickly pear and jojoba oil (if using).

5 / To the second bowl, add the rose, frankincense, and helichrysum essential oils.

6 / Add the contents of the second bowl to the cactus water mixture and stir.

7 / Apply to the face, avoiding the eyes and mouth, with a facial brush or clean fingers.

8 / Let sit for 15 to 20 minutes before rinsing off with warm water. Follow with toner and moisturizer.

9 / Refrigerate extra material in a clean jar with lid and use within 2 weeks.

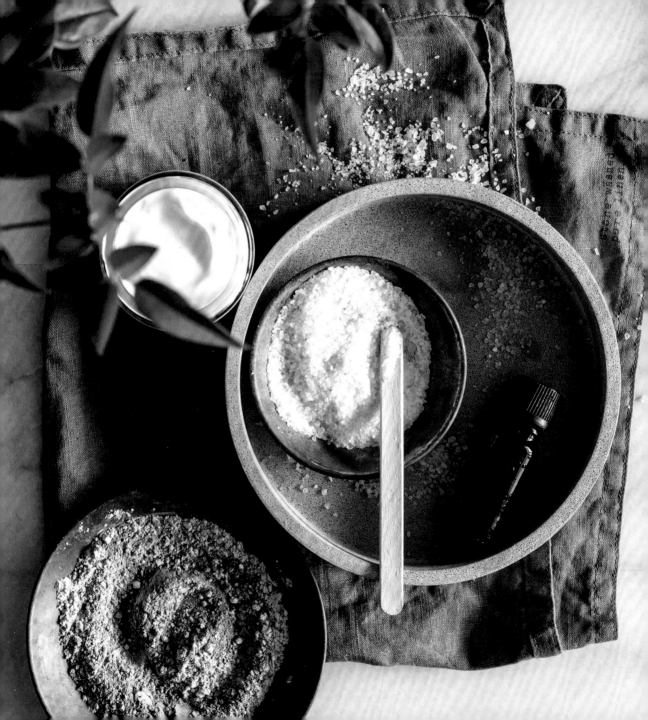

Dead Sea Mud Mask

The minerals found in mud and clay work wonders on skin, and I love to recreate their soft, glowing effects. Mud has been used in beauty recipes for centuries—and for good reason! Mud masks not only leave your face feeling soft and smooth, but leave skin aglow thanks to the increase in blood supply.

MATERIALS

1 teaspoon Dead Sea mineral salt

2 teaspoons clay

1 tablespoon plain yogurt

1 drop tea tree oil

1 / Pour the mineral salt and clay into a small, nonmetal bowl.

2 / Mix in yogurt and tea tree oil.

3 / Slowly add warm water until the consistency of the mask is smooth and spreadable. Depending on the brand and thickness of your yogurt, the amount of water needed may vary.

4 / Apply to your face and neck, avoiding the eye area.

5 / Leave on for 10 to 15 minutes before rinsing with warm water.

TIP
All skin types can benefit from mud, but if you're not sure which clay to use in this recipe, bentonite clay works well for most skin types. If your skin is super sensitive, stick with a gentle clay like white kaolin or French green.

Champagne + Clay Detox Face Mask

If you need a little detoxifying, then a champagne-based facial mask is perfect for the job. This anti-inflammatory treatment will pull toxins from your skin, while the antioxidants from the champagne will soothe the skin and give it a lovely glow—so let's pop that champagne open and get masking!

MATERIALS

4 ounces (113 g) powdered clay (bentonite is a great choice for all skin types)

2 tablespoons heavy cream, half-and-half, or plain yogurt

¼ cup champagne

1 / Pour the powdered clay into a mixing bowl.

2 / Slowly add in the cream—if you are using heavy cream or yogurt with a high fat content, you might want to reduce the amount—gently mixing it with the clay as you pour.

3 / Once that's done, add in the champagne, mixing the mask the entire time.

4 / Apply to face and neck and let sit for 15 to 20 minutes.

5 / Once the mask has dried, rinse with warm water and a washcloth.

TIP
This mask can be done once every week or two as overall skin health maintenance, preferably right before your normal daily or nightly skincare routine.

Anti-Inflammatory Spirulina + Avocado Face Mask

Combining spirulina with avocado makes a skin-soothing face mask that evens out skin tone and calms skin irritation. Spirulina, a blue-green algae, is a rich source of antioxidants, which help reduce inflammation and prevent skin damage. It's also rich in bioactive compounds that fight bacteria, which can help with acne. So let this green goodness make your skin truly glow.

MATERIALS

½ avocado

2 spirulina capsules, or 1 teaspoon bulk spirulina powder

1 teaspoon avocado oil

TOOLS

Facial brush (optional)

1 / Put the avocado in a bowl and mash with a fork until it has a smooth consistency. Mash thoroughly, because the smoother the avocado is, the easier it will be to apply the mask to your face.

2 / When the avocado is super smooth, without any lumps or bumps, add the spirulina and avocado oil and stir to combine.

3 / Mix until well blended—you'll be able to tell because the mask will be an even blue-green, thanks to the spirulina.

4 / Apply the mask to clean skin with your fingers or a facial brush. You'll want a nice, even layer.

5 / Leave the mask on for 15 minutes and remove with warm water. Pat skin dry and apply toner and moisturizer.

NOTE This is a great mask to follow up any exfoliation. It's hydrating and replenishes lost moisture, for glowing, healthy skin. And even better: No more avocados left to the sad fate of turning brown in the fridge!

ALOE VERA MASKS FOR EVERY SKIN TYPE

Aloe vera is anti-inflammatory, cell renewing, and fantastic for all skin types. It moisturizes without clogging pores, so even the oiliest of skins can benefit—really, aloe should be in every beauty routine.

FOR MATURE SKIN

The antioxidants in blueberries brighten dull skin, while the coffee reduces puffiness.

6 to 8 blueberries

1 teaspoon aloe vera gel

½ teaspoon finely ground coffee

In a small bowl, mash the blueberries then add the aloe vera gel and coffee. Refrigerate for 1 hour. Gently apply, then rinse with warm water after 15 minutes.

SOOTHE SUNBURN

Aloe vera is a sunburn classic—not just an anti-inflammatory, it also stimulates collagen production to help skin repair. Raw honey is another natural healer.

1 tablespoon aloe vera gel

1 tablespoon raw honey

Store-bought aloe is fine, but so is gel from the plant! Pop it in a blender to get a smooth consistency. Combine ingredients and apply to face and any other sunburned areas.

FOR DEHYDRATED SKIN

Avocado face masks are super soothing for dry, dehydrated skin. The healthy fat in avocado helps maintain moisture, while the omega-fatty acids soothe irritation.

¼ mashed avocado

1 tablespoon aloe vera gel

1 tablespoon oats

Mix all ingredients together well. For a smoother mask, grind up the oats using a coffee grinder or food processor. Apply to face and leave for 10 to 15 minutes before rinsing with warm water.

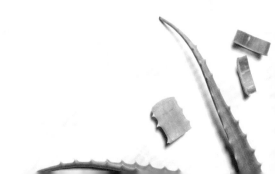

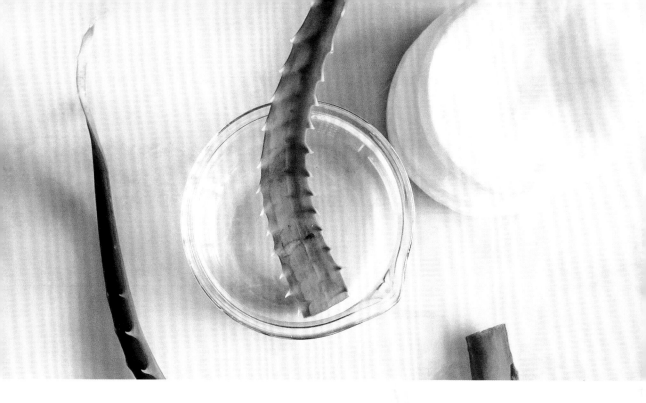

FOR ACNE-PRONE SKIN 1

Tea tree oil is a highly potent skincare ingredient that doesn't just banish acne—it's antibacterial and anti-inflammatory, so it zaps the zits at the source.

4 tablespoons aloe vera gel

1 drop tea tree oil (more may be irritating, so don't overdo it)

½ peeled cucumber

Blend ingredients well and apply to face with fingertips or facial brush. Leave on for 10 to 15 minutes, then rinse.

FOR ACNE-PRONE SKIN 2

Charcoal absorbs excess oil, while aloe is soothing and anti-inflammatory, making it ideal for acne.

1 tablespoon activated charcoal

1 tablespoon aloe vera gel

1 drop of tea tree oil

Combine ingredients in a bowl and mix together with fingers before applying. In circular motions, work the charcoal mixture around your face for 1 minute, then let sit for 10 to 15 minutes. Rinse thoroughly with warm water.

Acne & Oily Skin

My mom used to tell my teenaged self that in 20 years I'd be thankful for my oily skin. Maybe she was right, but in the meantime? It can be a serious cause for annoyance! With lots of oil and shine, you feel the need to wash your face more often, but harsh scrubs and cleansers can irritate the skin and overstimulate your pores to produce even more oil, creating a frustrating cycle. And then there's acne, which has no silver linings at all.

Sometimes you need a little extra assistance in getting rid of the excess oil, dead skin cells, and dirt clogging your pores. That's what these masks are for. Whether they're reducing oil or dealing with blackheads and acne at the source, these masks will help your skin glow—rather than shine.

Nutmeg Spot Treatment Mask

Combine these three acne fighters to shrink a pimple fast—without leaving your skin dry or flaky.

MATERIALS

1 aspirin tablet, not enteric-coated

¼ teaspoon nutmeg

1 tablespoon plain yogurt

1 / Crush the aspirin tablet down into a powder and place the results in a small bowl.

2 / Add the nutmeg and yogurt and stir to make a paste.

3 / Gently dab on the zit.

4 / Leave on for 10 to 15 minutes, then rinse with warm water.

Honey + Baking Soda Mask

Baking soda is just one of those things that everyone should have because it is incredibly useful for so many different things—including beauty. Adding baking soda to your skincare routine can reduce skin irritation and itching, plus provide detoxifying benefits.

MATERIALS

1 teaspoon lemon juice

1 tablespoon honey

1 teaspoon baking soda

1 / Add lemon juice, honey, and baking soda to a small bowl.

2 / Mix well until the texture is smooth and even.

3 / Apply over your face and neck. Avoid the area near your eyes—both lemon juice and honey will sting. Don't turn this into a scrub by rubbing it into your skin.

4 / After 15 minutes, remove the mask with warm water, then rinse with cold water.

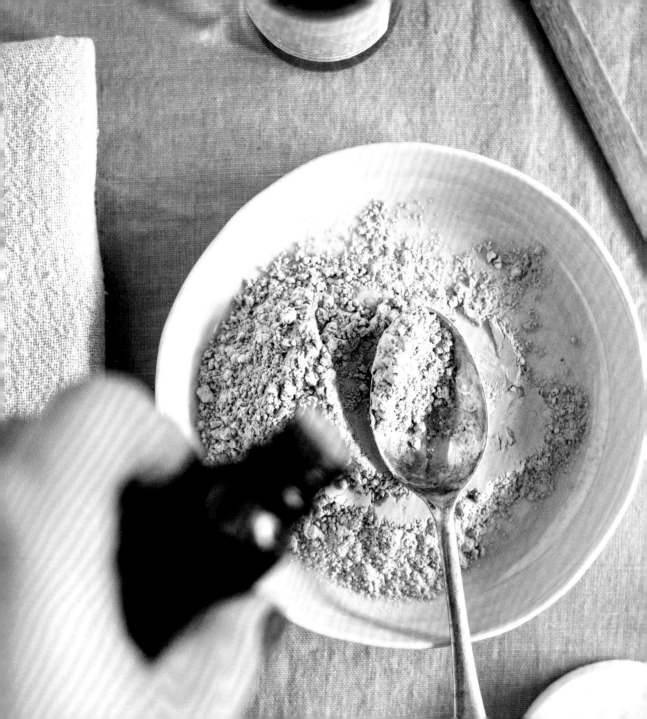

Apple Cider Vinegar + Clay Face Mask

Clay draws out impurities in the pores, while the natural acids in apple cider vinegar address acne by gently sloughing away dead skin cells.

MATERIALS

1 tablespoon bentonite clay

1 probiotic capsule

2 tablespoons raw apple cider vinegar

1 / Combine clay and probiotic powder in a small bowl.

2 / Add the apple cider vinegar and stir to make a paste. It's okay to use more, if needed, to get a smooth, spreadable consistency.

3 / With clean fingers, spread the mask over your face and let sit for 15 minutes.

4 / Rinse with cool water and apply moisturizer.

Witch Hazel Sheet Mask

Sheet masks are super fun and on-trend—but buying too many of them can really break the bank. So make your own DIY sheet masks with a simple tissue! After all, the sheet is simply a vehicle to transport the fluids or ingredients to the skin.

Tea tree's antibacterial properties are a great addition to any sheet mask—especially for those battling acne—while witch hazel is also wonderful for calming inflammation and redness.

MATERIALS

¼ cup distilled water

2 drops tea tree oil

¼ cup witch hazel

TOOLS

Tissues

1 / Combine the water, tea tree oil, and witch hazel in a bowl and mix well.

2 / Cut or tear the tissue in half at the fold, so you have two pieces, for the top and bottom halves of your face.

3 / Place the tissue halves into the bowl to absorb the liquid.

4 / Once fully saturated, remove from the liquid and simply put on your face to apply.

5 / Leave the sheets on for 10 to 15 minutes, then remove and gently dab off any excess liquid.

6 / Rinsing is optional for this mask, but follow with appropriate serum or moisturizer.

Potato Green Tea Overnight Mask

Wearing a healing mask all night allows our skin the chance to heal and repair cells, balance oil production, and expel impurities. This skin renewal process is part of what makes overnight masks so wonderfully beneficial—like this one, which takes advantage of the anti-inflammatory properties of potato juice and the antioxidants and antibacterial agents in green tea.

MATERIALS

1 tablespoon raw potato juice

1 tablespoon green tea

TOOLS

Cotton pads

TIP

These masks can get a little messy! If you want to avoid staining your favorite set of sheets, have an old pillowcase—preferably a dark one—handy to use on these nights.

1 / Take a clean, washed potato and juice it to extract 1 tablespoon of potato juice.

2 / Steep 2 bags of green tea in hot water for 10 minutes, then set aside to cool.

3 / Once cool, remove 1 tablespoon of green tea from the cup and mix it with the potato juice.

4 / Dip a cotton pad in the solution and apply to a clean face, taking your time to apply to any clogged areas or blemishes.

5 / In the morning, use your normal facial cleanser and follow with your daily skincare routine.

Garlic + Milk Mask

Garlic works to prevent clogged pores, kill off acne-causing bacteria, and reduce inflammation. Garlic can sting if applied directly to the skin, so dilute it with milk, honey, or aloe vera gel. Jojoba hydrates without clogging pores, while whole milk gently exfoliates.

MATERIALS

1 clove garlic, crushed and finely minced

1 teaspoon jojoba oil

2 tablespoons whole milk, honey, or aloe vera gel

1 / Combine garlic and jojoba oil in a small bowl.

2 / Slowly add the milk (or honey or aloe), stirring until you have a smooth consistency.

3 / Wear the mask for 5 to 10 minutes, then gently massage the skin as you rinse with warm water.

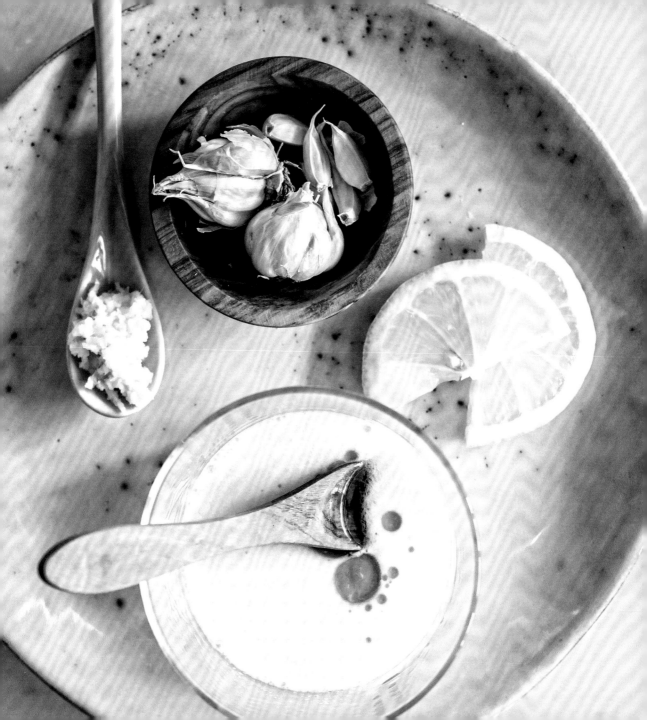

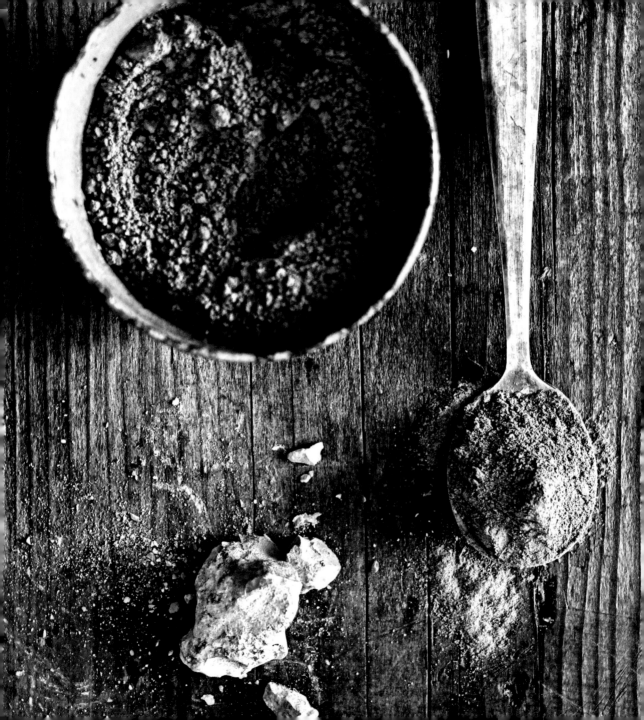

Moroccan Red Clay + Rosewater Mask

Moroccan red clay is an ideal choice for balancing oily skin and unclogging pores. It absorbs excess oil and is often used in recipes for deodorants and masks. Mined in the mountains of Morocco, this clay deep cleanses the pores while stimulating circulation—yet it's still gentle enough for sensitive skin.

MATERIALS

3 tablespoons rosewater

1 teaspoon mashed avocado

2 tablespoons Moroccan red clay

1 / Make your own rosewater using the recipe on page 53.

2 / Be sure avocado is thoroughly mashed.

3 / Combine the rosewater, avocado, and clay in a bowl and stir thoroughly.

4 / Keep mixing until a smooth paste is created and all the clay has been incorporated into the mixture.

5 / Using clean fingers or a facial brush, apply mask to the T-zone or acne-prone areas.

6 / As soon as the mask starts to lighten (usually a sign the mask is dry), rinse off with warm water.

TIP
The monounsaturated fat in the avocado will help nourish all skin types, and balance oil too.

Pigmentation Changes

With aging comes those frustrating dark spots on your face and body. But aging isn't the only cause for spots—excessive sun exposure is often a culprit, too. That's why sun protection is, of course, the most important part of preventing pigmentation changes. But let's be honest—we're all sometimes a little less good about using sunscreen than we should be. Luckily, even though you may have overdone it in the sun for several years, there are still ways to reduce the appearance of unwanted scars, age spots and other discolorations. And that's good, because no matter how much prevention you do, sun exposure and aging are a part of life. So let these brightening treatments go to work to even out skin tone, help fade dark spots, and reveal fresher looking skin.

Fuller's Earth + Honey + Rosewater Mask

A sedimentary clay, fuller's Earth has lightening properties that help with pigmentation changes and aging skin. Due to its strength, fuller's earth can also be combined with small amounts of bentonite clay. Receiving its name from textile workers called fullers, who used this clay to remove oil from wool, this has become a choice clay for drawing out excess sebum and decolorizing (lightening) oil out of pores.

MATERIALS

1 tablespoon rosewater

2 teaspoons fuller's earth

1 teaspoon honey

1 / Make your own rosewater using the recipe on page 53.

2 / Pour the fuller's earth clay and rosewater into a small, nonmetal bowl.

3 / Add in the honey and blend thoroughly.

4 / Apply 1 to 2 times a week for 10 minutes.

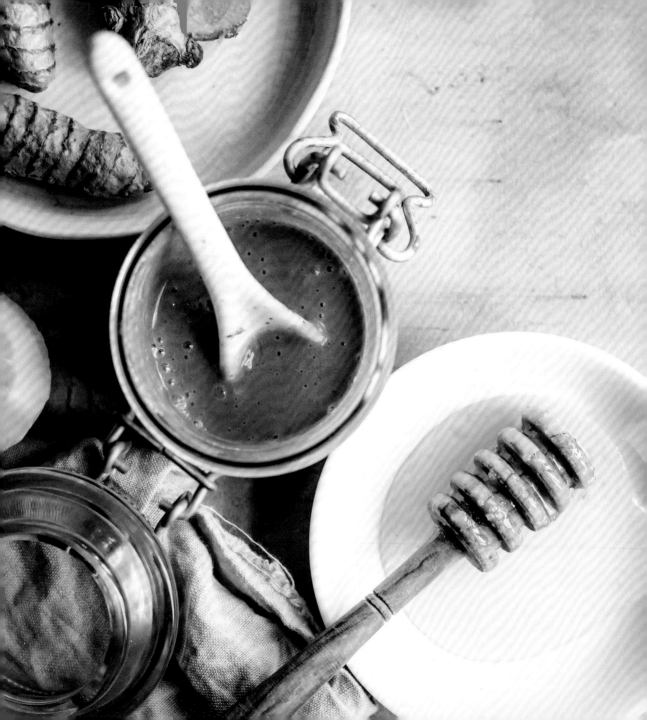

Turmeric Mask

Turmeric has been popping up in beauty products for centuries, and for good reason. Simply combine turmeric with a little coconut milk and honey and voila! An anti-inflammatory, anti-aging turmeric face mask that will leave you with glowing skin. And the best part is that this turmeric mask works its de-puffing magic in just 10 minutes!

MATERIALS

1½ teaspoons ground turmeric

1 teaspoon raw organic honey

1 tablespoon coconut milk

1 to 2 drops orange essential oil

1 / Put turmeric, honey, and coconut milk into a small bowl and stir.

2 / Add the orange essential oil and stir again.

3 / You want your mask to be a thin paste, so adjust the coconut milk as necessary until you get the right consistency.

4 / Apply the mask evenly all over your face, being sure to focus on any inflamed areas.

5 / Leave the mask on for 20 minutes, then rinse off with warm water.

Honey + Spirulina Face Mask

Whether you're fighting dandruff or looking for a formidable opponent to fight free radicals, inflammation, and aging, spirulina just might be your dream come true. The amount of antioxidants found in spirulina is four times the amount found in berries! It can also help boost skin tone and complexion and leave you with that sought-after, dewy glow.

MATERIALS

1 tablespoon organic honey

1 tablespoon spirulina powder

1 / Mix the honey and spirulina powder together to form a paste.

2 / Apply to your face and neck with fingertips or a facial brush.

3 / Leave the mask on for 20 minutes, then rinse off with warm water and a washcloth.

4 / Once the entire mask is removed, follow with a moisturizer or serum for added hydration.

TIP
Be sure to check with your doctor if you're currently on any prescriptions, as spirulina can occasionally interfere with medication.

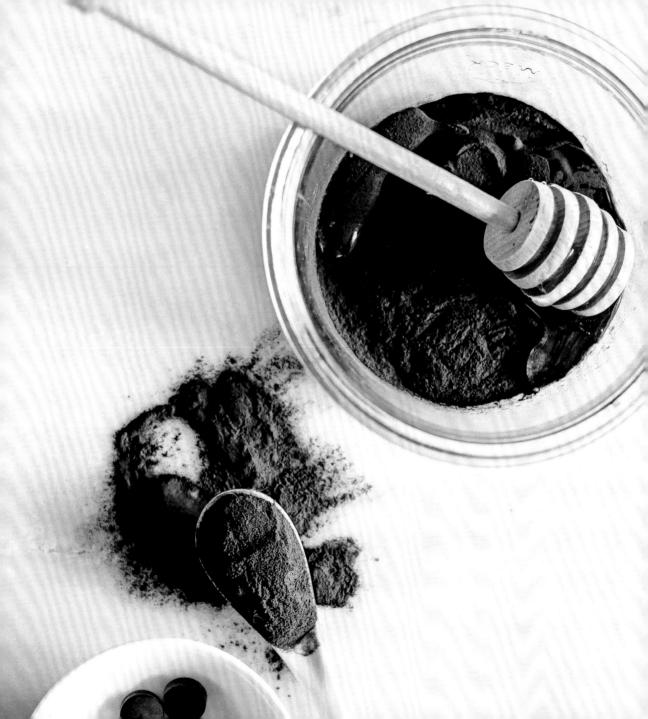

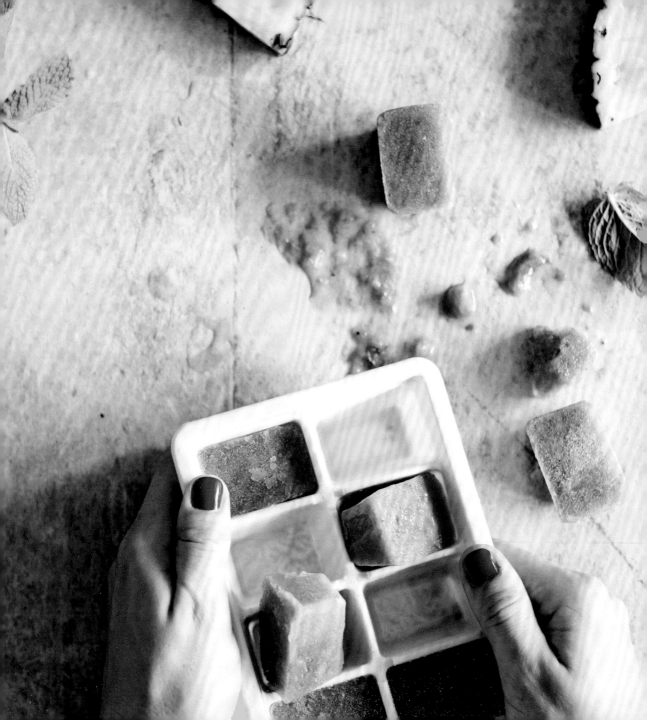

Tropical Enzyme Ice Mask

This tropical enzyme-packed mask is great for aging skin, pigmentation problems, and overall exfoliation. Packed full of potent vitamins and compounds, this mask will help dissolve dead skin cells while moisturizing ones that remain. It's a great mask for year-round use.

MATERIALS

½ fresh papaya, peeled and seeded

1 cup pineapple

5 strawberries

1 tablespoon honey

TOOLS

Blender

Ice cube tray

1 / Peel and seed the papaya.

2 / In a blender, combine all ingredients and blend until pureed.

3 / There is usually enough water in the fruit to let it puree well, but if you need to add a little water, go ahead.

4 / Apply some to your face immediately, avoiding the eye area, and pour into ice cube trays whatever does not get used immediately and freeze for a later date.

5 / Whenever you would like a mask, pop out a cube and defrost by placing in a bowl and leaving it on the counter until soft.

6 / You can mash the cube with a fork as it softens and then apply with fingertips, avoiding the eye area. Leave on for 10 minutes, then rinse with warm water and follow with moisturizer.

Dark Chocolate Honey Mask

Chocolate—just saying the word makes my mouth water. I love all things chocolate, from rich brownies and cakes to decadent truffles and nuts drenched in melted chocolate goodness.

Chocolate contains plentiful antioxidants that protect your skin and help reduce lines and wrinkles. But not all chocolate is created equal—for health and beauty, dark chocolate is the best.

MATERIALS

3 to 5 squares dark chocolate

2 teaspoons ground oats

⅛ cup honey

1 tablespoon plain Greek yogurt

TOOLS

Small pot or saucepan

Heat-proof bowl

Coffee grinder

TIP
Try to purchase chocolate with a high cacao content—at least 70 percent!

1 / Add 2 to 3 inches of water to the small pot or saucepan and place the bowl on top, so that it's not touching the water.

2 / Heat the water to a simmer, then turn off the heat and add about half of the chocolate to the bowl and stir to melt.

3 / Stir in the remaining chocolate a little bit at a time, and mix until it's all melted.

4 / Remove the bowl from the pot and set on the counter to cool.

5 / Grind oatmeal in a coffee grinder, enough to get 2 teaspoons of ground oats.

6 / Pour the honey, yogurt, and ground oats, into the chocolate and mix the ingredients into a smooth, creamy paste.

7 / Massage the mask into your face with your fingers, using gentle, circular motions.

8 / Leave the mask on for 15 minutes, then rinse thoroughly with warm water.

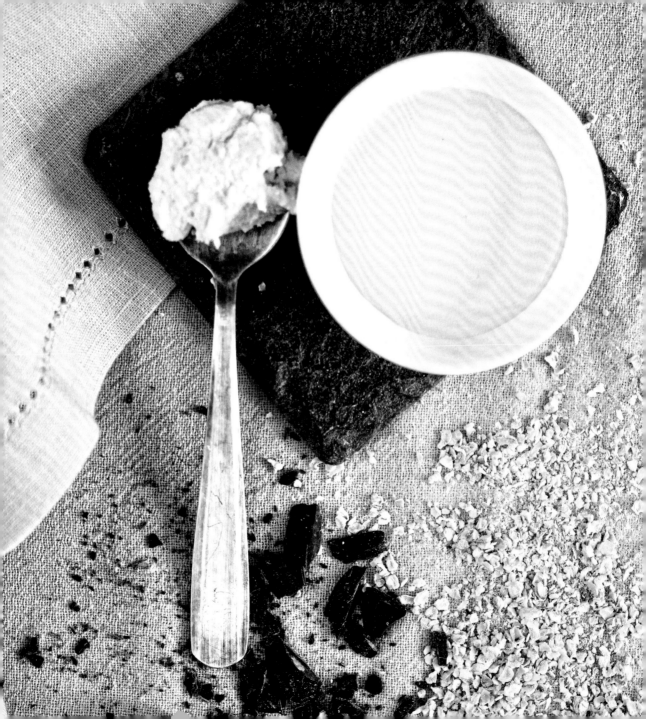

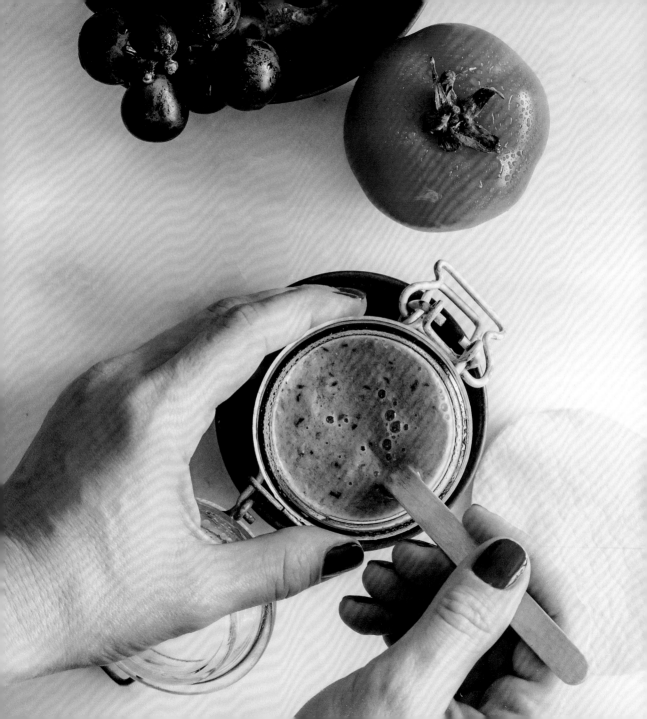

Pigmentation Grape Face Mask

The lightening properties of tomatoes and grapes make this mask a powerful duo that fights age spots and sun damage, while overall evening out complexions. And if that wasn't enough, The polyphenol resveratrol found in the skin of red grapes can increase collagen production and neutralize free-radical damage.

MATERIALS

¼ tomato

5 to 6 red grapes

1 / In a blender, pulse the tomato and grapes, creating a wet paste.

2 / Apply to face and neck, concentrating on any sun spots or darker areas.

3 / Leave on for 20 minutes before rinsing thoroughly.

CLAY MASKS
FOR EVERY SKIN TYPE

Clay can work wonders on a wide range of skin conditions, and bentonite clay is particularly flexible. Important note: Never use metal with clay—use glass or wooden instruments instead.

FOR DRY SKIN

Nourish and hydrate your skin with this lovely mask—and its rosy scent.

1 tablespoon bentonite clay

1 tablespoon rosehip oil

1 tablespoon rosewater

1 drop essential oil*

Combine ingredients in a bowl, using enough rosewater to make a smooth paste. Apply and let sit for 15 minutes. Rinse with cool water.

*Essential oils for dry skin: geranium, sandalwood, palmarosa, myrrh, patchouli, Roman chamomile

FOR MATURE SKIN 1

Orange juice is loaded with vitamin C, one of the best weapons against free radicals, age spots, and uneven skin tone.

2 tablespoons fresh squeezed orange juice

1 tablespoon bentonite clay

1 teaspoon raw honey

Combine ingredients and mix until you have a smooth consistency, adding more juice if needed. Apply evenly, avoiding the eyes. Relax for 10 to 15 minutes, then rinse.

FOR SENSITIVE SKIN

Cocoa powder delivers tons of antioxidants to help repair damaged skin. Look for plain dark chocolate with a 70 percent or higher cocoa content.

1 tablespoon kaolin clay

1 tablespoon cocoa powder

Combine ingredients and stir. Add enough water to make a smooth paste. Apply, relax for 15 minutes, and remove.

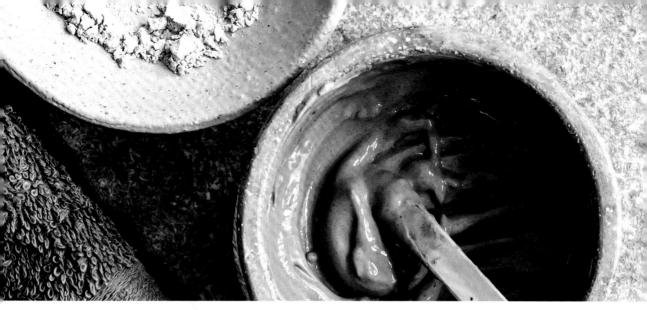

FOR ACNE-PRONE SKIN

This mask combines bentonite clay with the purifying, absorbent power of activated charcoal and the benefits of probiotics.

1 tablespoon bentonite clay

1 tablespoon activated charcoal

1 probiotic capsule

2 tablespoons raw apple cider vinegar

1 drop essential oil*

Combine ingredients and stir to make a paste. Add more apple cider vinegar if needed to make smooth. Apply and let sit for 15 minutes. Rinse with cool water.

*Essential oils for acne: tea tree, juniper berry, lavender, cedarwood, lemon, cypress

FOR MATURE SKIN 2

Green tea and vitamin C both provide powerful antioxidant protection, essential to slowing the effects of aging.

1 tablespoon bentonite clay

½ teaspoon vitamin C powder

2 tablespoons green tea, cooled

1 drop essential oil*

Combine ingredients in a small bowl. Add enough green tea to make a smooth paste. Apply and let sit for 15 minutes. Rinse with cool water.

*Essential oils for wrinkles: rose, sandalwood, helichrysum, frankincense, rose geranium

Mature Skin

Does anyone really know the secret to slowing the aging process? As my age creeps higher, I find myself paying more attention to anti-aging facts and solutions. I don't mind getting older, but I certainly don't want to suddenly look (or feel) it! Feeling comfortable and confident in your own skin is definitely the most important factor in aging well.

Chances are you're also doing all you can to maintain youthful looking skin—and keep in mind, age prevention is most effective if it starts when you're young! Maybe you're diligent about wearing sunscreen, using anti-aging products, and guzzling water. But sometimes you just want that little extra boost—so here are some fun masks to help you age well and maintain your gorgeous glow.

Firming Aloe Vera Mask for Mature Skin

Carrots are a rich source of beta-carotene, a skin-friendly form of vitamin A that supports healthier, younger-looking skin, and protects against sun exposure and even pollution.

That's why it's so crucial to use a regular carrot instead of the baby ones. Baby carrots lose a lot of their natural nutrients when turned into little nubs, while whole carrots are still packed full of all the things that are good for you—inside and out.

MATERIALS

1 egg white

1 tablespoon finely shredded carrot

1 teaspoon aloe vera gel

TOOLS

Facial brush (optional)

1 / Combine egg white, carrot, and aloe vera in a small bowl.

2 / Beat the mixture together with a fork until frothy, which should take about a minute.

3 / With clean hands or a facial brush, apply the mask to the face and eye area.

4 / Let the mask dry for 15 to 30 minutes.

5 / Rinse with warm water and follow with moisturizer.

TIP
You may feel the mask tightening your skin, but if it gets uncomfortable, go ahead and remove it early. Remove with warm water.

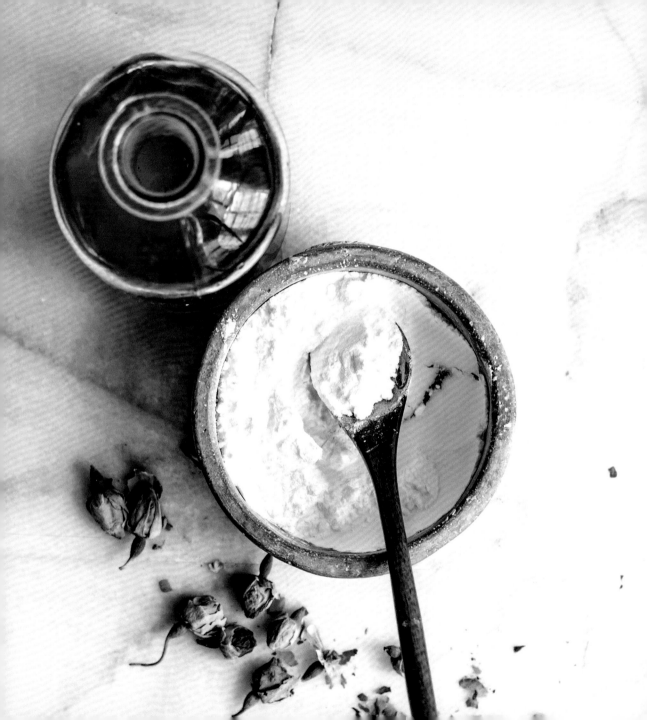

Pearl Powder Mask

There's no shortage of weird ingredients to put on your face. Mud. Snail slime. And . . . pearls? Yes, pearls! Adding those to your skin regime might sound pricey, but you don't need a Kardashian-sized budget to afford pearl beauty treatments.

Yes, pearl powder really is powder made from pearls, just like those found in jewelry. Freshwater pearls are ground into a super fine powder that's easily absorbed and used by the body. Used externally, pearls gently exfoliate, accelerate skin metabolism to tone and rejuvenate skin, fade blemishes, reduce pores, and decrease redness. Plus, you'll get to feel like a queen.

MATERIALS

2 to 3 teaspoons rosewater

1 teaspoon pearl powder

1 / Make yourself some rosewater (see recipe on page 53).

2 / Mix the pearl powder and rosewater together and stir to make a paste.

3 / Apply to face, as well as chest or hands if desired.

4 / Leave on for 15 minutes and then rinse with warm water. The mask can be drying, so follow with moisturizer and only use 1 to 2 times per week.

Berry + Yogurt Age-Fighting Mask

Blackberries are extremely high in antioxidants, as well as vitamins A, C, and K. They fight free radicals that lead to premature aging, and are a wonderful ingredient for a facial mask. Combine their antioxidant power with yogurt's gentle exfoliating properties, and you've got a match—I mean mask—made in heaven.

MATERIALS

2 tablespoons organic plain yogurt

2 tablespoons raw organic honey

¼ cup blackberries or mixed berries

TOOLS

Blender

Facial brush

1 / Combine yogurt, honey, and berries in a blender.

2 / Pulse blender until the mixture is smooth.

3 / Apply the mask to clean skin with facial brush and leave on for 10 to 20 minutes.

4 / Rinse off with warm water and follow with moisturizer.

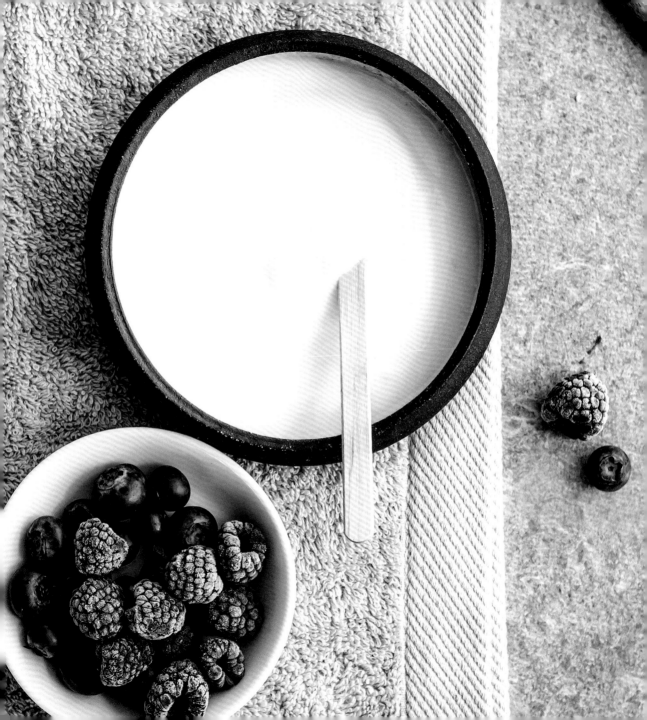

Cranberry + Clay Brightening Mask

Filled with antioxidants and B vitamins, cranberries provide a powerful shield against pollutant factors and are fantastic for brightening dull, lackluster skin. These dark red fruits are also high in vitamin C, which helps keep skin firm by boosting collagen production and slowing down the aging process. And of course, their vivid color makes this mask a visual delight.

MATERIALS

¼ cup cranberries

¼ teaspoon Rhassoul clay

1 teaspoon plain Greek yogurt

1 teaspoon honey

¼ cup water (or as needed)

TOOLS

Blender

1 / Start by blending the cranberries until they are pasty in texture.

2 / In a bowl, combine the blended cranberries, Rhassoul clay, yogurt, and honey.

3 / To make the cream thinner, mix in water slowly until it reaches your desired consistency. You'll want the mask to be easy to apply, but not so watery it slides off your face.

4 / Leave on your face for 10 to 15 minutes and then rinse thoroughly with warm water to remove.

Egg White + Honey + Oat Mask

Bring the comfort of a warm, hearty breakfast to your skincare with this wonderful mask. This mask covers so many bases, from tightening skin to exfoliating to skin healing—and even better, it's so simple to make.

MATERIALS

1 egg white

1 teaspoon honey

1 to 2 tablespoons ground oats or flour

1 / Whip together the egg white and honey until well combined and a bit frothy.

2 / Add ground oats or flour and stir until you have a paste.

3 / Apply to face, avoiding the eyes, and massage the paste gently into your skin.

4 / Leave mask on for 10 minutes and remove with warm water.

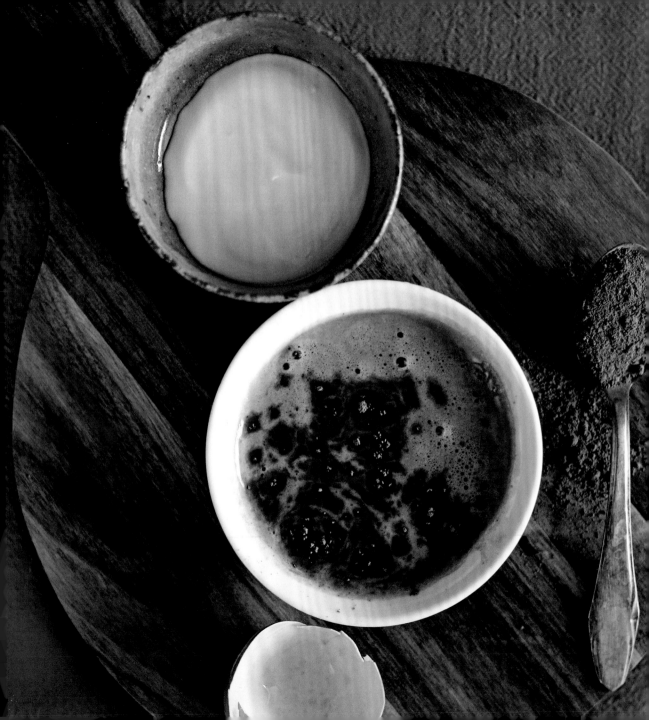

Cocoa + Cream Mask

Alpha hydroxy acids rapidly exfoliate the skin, revealing fresh, new skin cells and evening out skin tone. There are a lot of products containing AHAs out there today, but natural AHA masks can be easily created at home with just a few fresh ingredients.

MATERIALS

1 tablespoon sour cream

1 tablespoon honey

1 tablespoon cocoa powder

1 egg white

1 / Combine the sour cream and honey in a bowl, mixing thoroughly.

2 / Stir in the cocoa powder and egg white.

3 / Keep stirring until a smooth, even texture is attained.

4 / Apply to the face and neck, and leave the mask on until it dries.

5 / Rinse with warm water to remove. Follow with your usual moisturizer.

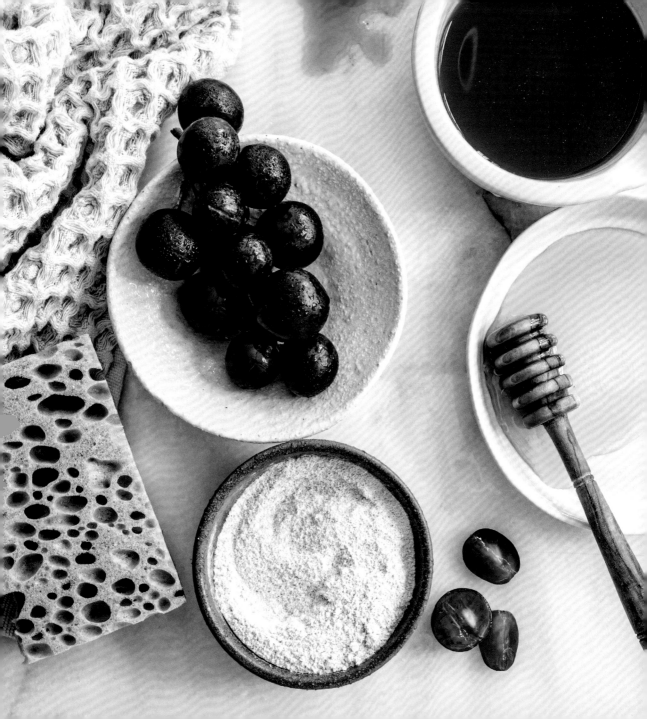

Wrinkle-Smoothing Wine Face Mask

An at-home facial is the perfect way to unwind after a long week. I highly recommend drawing a bath, mixing up a face mask, and relaxing with a glass of wine. Stress doesn't stand a chance. Inspired by the anti-aging properties of wine, this facial incorporates the antioxidants in grapes and wines to smooth wrinkles and fight free radicals for healthy, glowing skin.

MATERIALS

1 tablespoon white kaolin clay

1 teaspoon honey

2 tablespoons wine, red or white

5 to 7 grapes

1 / Combine clay, honey, and wine together in a nonmetal bowl.

2 / Squeeze the grapes to add their fresh juice.

3 / Mix until you have a smooth consistency, adding more wine if needed.

4 / Spread the paste evenly over a clean face and neck, avoiding the eye area.

5 / Relax and let the mask penetrate for 10 to 15 minutes. Rinse and follow with moisturizer.

TIP
Pull together grapes, clay, and a bottle of wine, and invite a few friends over for a full night of pampering!

EGG WHITE MASKS FOR EVERY SKIN TYPE

Eggs whites are nutritional powerhouses. From aging skin to oily skin, they help with everything from firming to closing pores. Just be careful of egg allergies, and to avoid salmonella, make sure to keep out of your eyes and mouth.

FOR MATURE SKIN

Here, egg whites and green tea team up to tighten skin and battle the free radicals that age our skin.

½ cup green tea

1 egg white

1 tablespoon honey

Brew the green tea and let it cool to room temperature. In a small bowl, whisk the egg white until frothy, then stir in the tea and honey. Soak a washcloth or a reusable sheet mask and apply for 15 minutes.

FOR EVERY SKIN TYPE

Crushing grapes releases grapeseed oil, which is high in vitamin E, moisturizes without feeling greasy, and is great for your skin.

1 egg white

6 to 7 fresh, seeded grapes

Combine ingredients in a blender, blending until completely smooth to release the grapeseed oil. Once frothy, use a facial brush to apply the mask, using upward strokes. Leave on for 15 minutes, then rinse thoroughly.

PORE CLEANSING

The sugar will exfoliate the pores while the cornstarch absorbs any grime.

1 egg white

1 tablespoon white sugar

2 teaspoons cornstarch

Mix ingredients together and apply to your face. Let dry for 15 to 20 minutes, then peel off the mask very slowly. Rinse with warm water. Afterward, apply aloe vera to any sensitive areas.

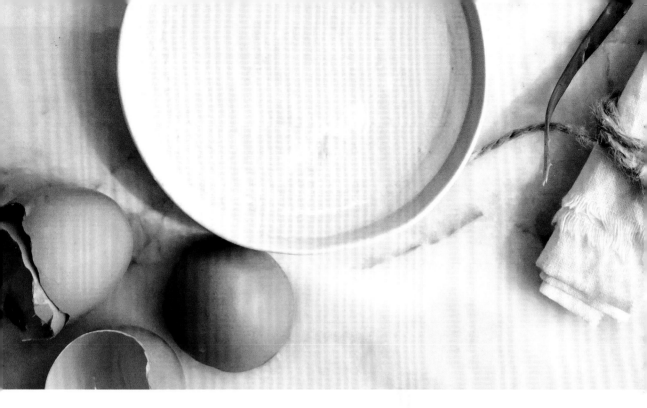

FOR OILY SKIN

Don't rush this one—you want the egg white to be fully dry so it can grab the gunk out of your pores for clear, blackhead-free skin!

1 egg white

Piece of tissue or toilet paper

Whip the egg white until frothy, then apply to your skin. Quickly lay the tissue on top and pat it to adhere with egg white. Keep it on until the egg is dry, then peel off and rinse with water.

FOR SENSITIVE SKIN

The aloe vera and chamomile tea soothe inflammation and redness on skin with slight irritation or inflammation—but don't use this mask on sunburns.

1 egg white

1 teaspoon aloe vera gel

1 teaspoon chamomile tea

Combine ingredients in a small bowl and whisk well. Apply and let dry for 20 minutes before rinsing with cool water.

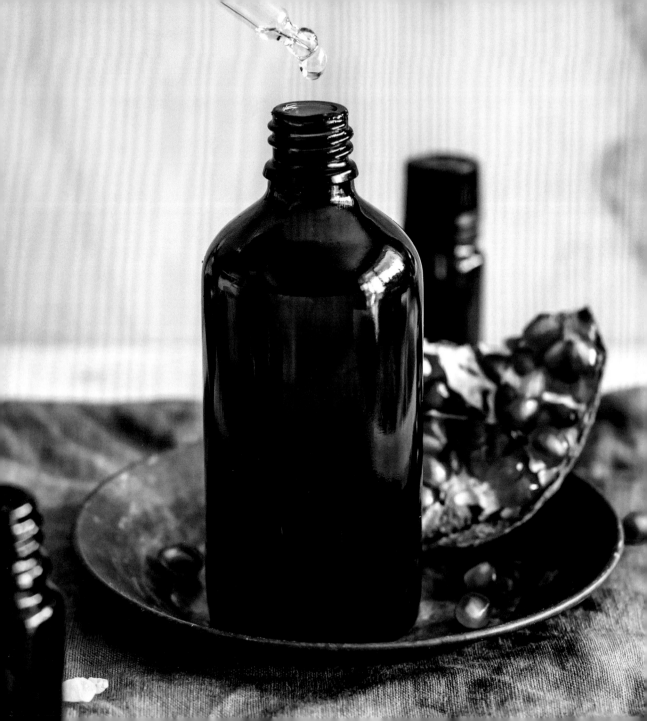

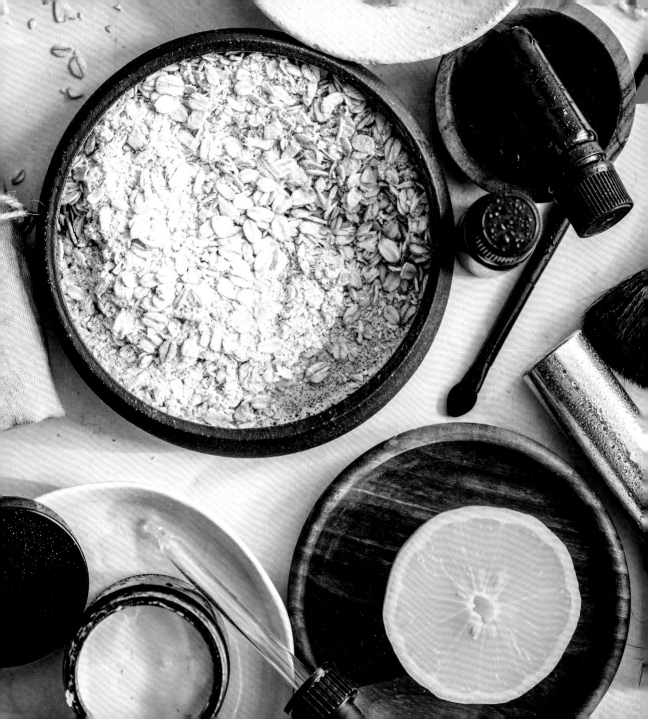

OVERNIGHT MASKS FOR EVERY SKIN TYPE

Think of overnight masks as intensive TLC for problem areas. Two warnings: Don't use them every night, so your skin can breathe. And these masks can get messy, so be sure to use old, dark pillowcases.

FOR DRY LIPS

Dry, chapped lips can be impossible to ignore—but this overnight mask is wonderful for healing them. Honey helps your skin retain moisture, and vitamin E treats the dry patches.

1 teaspoon vitamin E oil (about 3 vitamin E capsules)

1 teaspoon honey

Put the vitamin E oil—breaking open the capsules if necessary—and honey in a small bowl and mix thoroughly. Wear the mixture on your lips overnight and wipe off any excess in the morning.

FOR DRY SKIN

While this mask can be sticky, if you're looking for hydration, search no further.

1 teaspoon raw, unpasteurized honey

3 vitamin E capsules

¼ avocado

Combine ingredients in a bowl and mix well. Apply a thin layer to your face and neck at bedtime. In the morning, rinse the mask off thoroughly with warm water and a washcloth. Follow with your usual moisturizer and sunscreen.

FOR IRRITATION, ACNE, AND AGING

Combine the healing power of jojoba oil with the fragrant smell of rosewater in this soothing, anti-aging mask.

2 tablespoons rosewater

1 teaspoon jojoba oil

Combine ingredients and apply before bed. It's okay to apply over your evening moisturizer. And if you have oily skin, you can replace the jojoba oil with aloe vera gel. Rinse skin in the morning.

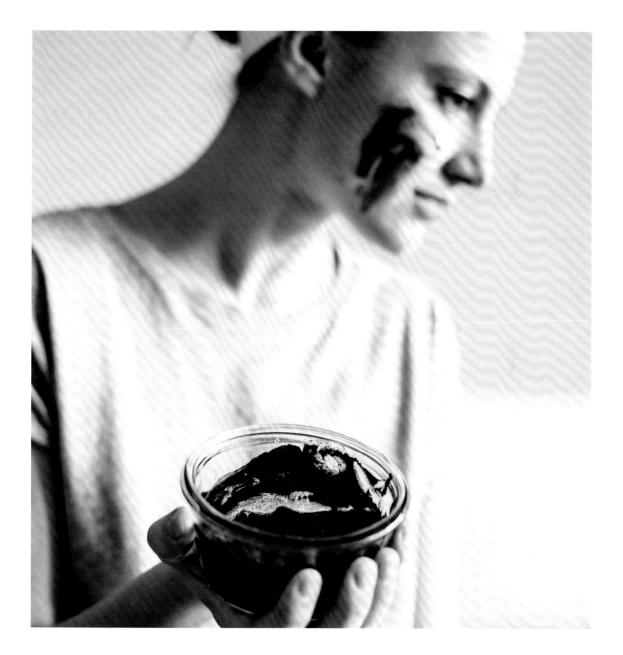

GORGEOUS ALL YEAR ROUND

Your skin changes with the cycle of the seasons, and so should your skincare! And since face masks target very specific issues, they're the perfect thing to adjust—and can give you the perfect seasonal vibes.

Spring

Cucumber Coconut Mask

While winter often leaves your skin feeling parched, this mask, spring, and fresh cucumber can all help it recover.

MATERIALS

1 cucumber

2 tablespoons coconut oil

½ teaspoon carrot seed oil

TOOLS

Blender

1 / Add ingredients to a blender and blend until creamy.

2 / Apply with facial brush or fingertips all over the face, neck, and eye area.

3 / Leave mask on for 10 to 15 minutes before washing off with warm water. Follow with moisturizer or serum.

Summer

Clear Skin Tomato Mask

Take advantage of summer produce for this skin-brightening mask, which helps with blotchy or uneven complexions.

MATERIALS

½ tomato

½ cucumber

2 tablespoons fresh parsley

TOOLS

Food processor

1 / Puree ingredients in a food processor until they reach a smooth consistency, about 1 minute.

2 / Apply mixture to clean skin, avoiding the eye area.

3 / Leave on for 10 minutes, then rinse with warm water and follow with a serum or moisturizer.

4 / Keep any leftovers in the fridge and use within 7 to 10 days.

Fall

Vitamin C Cranberry Facial Mask

This antioxidant-filled mask could only get better with a hot cup of cider and cozy blanket.

MATERIALS

7 to 9 fresh cranberries

1 teaspoon organic maple syrup

1 teaspoon plain organic yogurt

1 / Combine ingredients in small bowl.

2 / Use a fork to crush and whip in the cranberries.

3 / Apply at night with fingertips or a facial brush.

4 / Leave the mask on for 15 minutes before rinsing with warm water. Follow with moisturizer or serum.

Winter

Warming Paprika Mask

Keep yourself warm in the winter with this vibrant paprika mask, guaranteed to give a rosy glow.

MATERIALS

1 teaspoon paprika powder

Splash of goat milk (powdered goat milk can be used as substitute)

2 teaspoons raw honey

1 / Mix all ingredients well.

2 / Patch test on skin, especially if you're sensitive.

3 / Apply a thin layer to the face and neck, avoiding the eye area. Leave on for 5 minutes and remove with warm water and a washcloth. Follow with a serum or moisturizer.

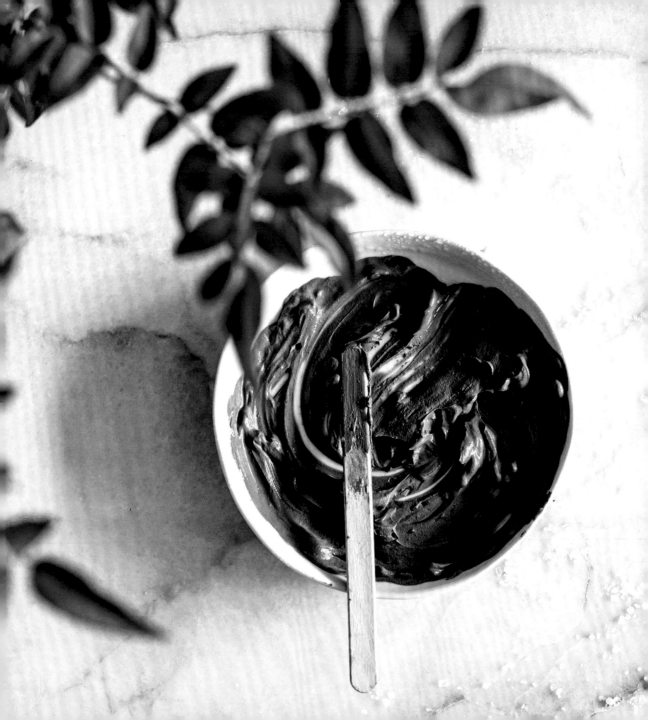

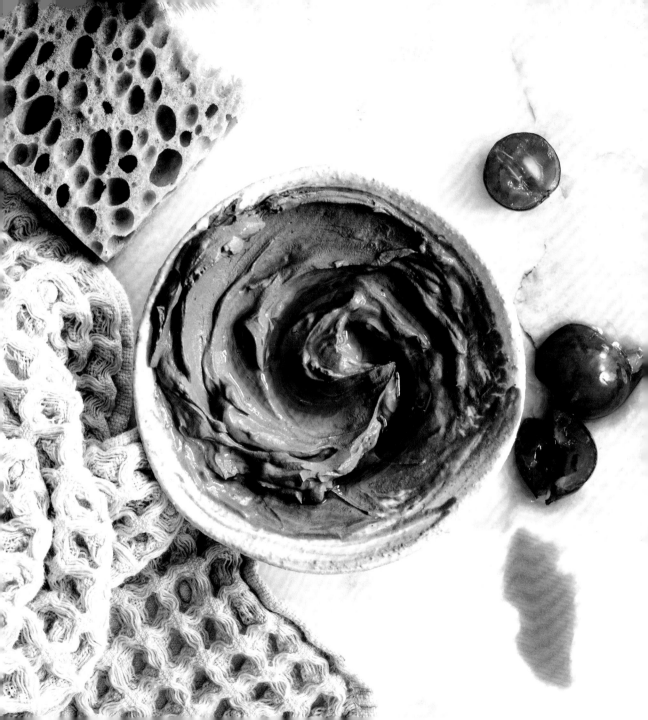

weldon**owen**

CEO Raoul Goff

Publisher Roger Shaw

Associate Publisher Mariah Bear

Creative Director Chrissy Kwasnik

Designer Leah Lauer

Produced by Weldon Owen
PO Box 3088
San Rafael, CA 94912
www.weldonowen.com
© 2020 Weldon Owen

ISBN 978-1-68188-575-9

Printed in Italy

10 9 8 7 6 5 4 3 2 1

2020 2021 2022 2023

Weldon Owen would like to thank Madeleine Calvi, Meagan Nolan, and Rachel Anderson for editorial assistance.

From the Author

The best part of Hello Glow is getting to work with such talented women. Thank you to Deborah Harju and Stephanie Pollard for creating recipes for the blog; I've learned so much from you both. I'm again in awe of Ana-Maria Stanciu's talent and feel so lucky to have her gorgeous photography in my books. I'm grateful for Dr. Gina Maria Jansheski for her insight and editing skills. And thank you to Daria Groza for sticking with me for the past crazy eight years, it's been quite a journey!

Photography

All photographs are by Ana-Maria Stanciu unless noted below:

Shutterstock: 12, 14, 28, 40, 86, 96, 120, 134, 138, 140, 142

Disclaimer

The recipes, products, and advice presented in this book do not guarantee results and should not be used for treating a serious health problem or disease. If you have any concerns about your skin or hair, consult your personal health practicioner before applying any recipe from this book. If you have sensitive skin, always do a patch test for any new products or treatments. The author's testimonials in this book represent anecdoctal experiences; individual experiences will vary. Neither the author nor the publisher may be held responsible for claims resulting from information in this book.